Your Grandmothers' Guide to Hispanic Folk Remedies & Advice

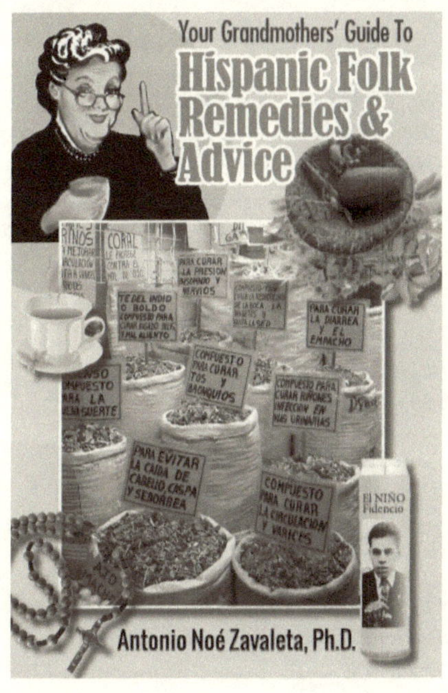

The Curandera's Household Healing Traditions of the Borderlands

Antonio Noé Zavaleta, Ph.D.

authorHOUSE

AuthorHouse™
1663 Liberty Drive
Bloomington, IN 47403
www.authorhouse.com
Phone: 833-262-8899

Published by AuthorHouse 02/02/2023

ISBN: 978-1-7283-7899-2 (sc)
ISBN: 979-8-8230-0000-0 (hc)
ISBN: 978-1-7283-7898-5 (e)

Includes bibliographical references and index

1. *Grandmother's Remedies and Advice*
2. *Curandera Spells*
3. *U.S.-Mexico Border Folklore & Health*
4. *Folk Medicine and Healing Traditions*
5. *Curanderismo*

An Important Note for my Readers

Your Grandmothers' Guide to Hispanic Remedies & *Advice*, is a book of Hispanic folklore not intended to serve as medical advice and is folklore for informational and educational purposes only.

Please note that there are many more remedies that are not included in this book, that would be impossible. Empty note pages at the back of the book are for you for jot down your memories.

Do not use the plants, remedies, practices or information described in this book for medical purposes. Please immediately contact a health-care professional about any condition that requires a diagnosis or medical attention.

Always consult a medical doctor first before considering or using any complementary or alternative health care material. The author and *Authorhouse* disclaim any liability arising directly or indirectly from the use of any of the plants or remedies or practices listed in this book.

Please also note that remedies are highly varied from culture to culture and from region to region so you will encounter many different remedies for a single ailment.

Acknowledgments

I thank my family who have supported and encouraged me throughout the time I have worked on this book, especially my wife Dr. Gabriela Sosa-Zavaleta and my son Michael Anthony Zavaleta.

The gift of time cannot ever be fully repaid. We especially thank remarkable *Curanderas* María Tamayo, Elisa Valle, †Josefa Contreras, †Jacinto Robles, †Don Perfecto Rodríguez, † Madre Panita and Manuel Robles for their faith and support over my 50-year journey in my study of *Curanderismo and Fidencismo*. A special thanks to my University of Texas anthropology professors †Don Americo Parades and Dr. Robert M. Malina as well as to author Jamie Sams a very special friend who has left us.

Special thanks and love for my two grandmothers, Conception Garcia Gomez and Mildred Linville Reid

The author wishes to acknowledge the special life-long contributions of Alberto Salinas, Jr.

Special recognition for graphic design by Gilbert Velasquez & Associates, Brownsville, Texas.

Table of Contents

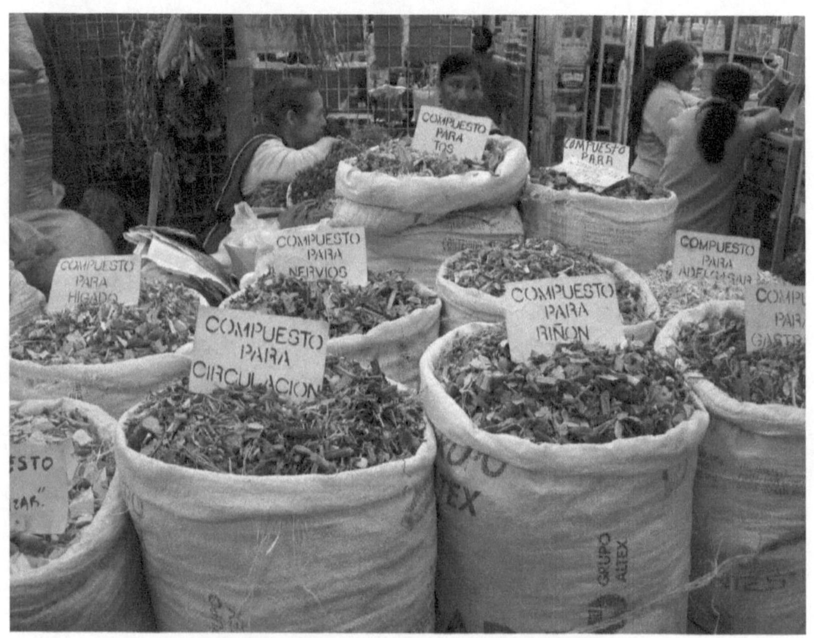

**Bulk medicinal plant sales at the
Mercado Sonora in Mexico City**

Introduction

Your Grandmothers' Guide to Hispanic Remedies & Advice: The Curanderas Household Healing Traditions of the Borderlands is a product of the *El Niño Fidencio Curanderismo Research Project*, property of and authored by anthropologist Antonio N. Zavaleta, Ph.D.

This ongoing *Curanderismo* research project was established in the 1970s, and operates the most comprehensive website on *Hispanic* folk healing and *Curanderismo available.* Search on the Internet for: **drzavaleta.com.**

The project utilizes time-honored methods in field anthropology, including ethnography and video-ethnography; participant observation-based field work in Espinazo, Nuevo León, México, as well as many other locations in Mexico and throughout the United States-Mexico border and the Caribbean.

As the lead anthropologist and project director Dr. Zavaleta has studied *Curanderismo* along the United States-Mexico border and The Fidencista Movement for more than 50 years.

Your Grandmothers' Guide to Hispanic Remedies & Advice serves to assist the average person to understand what *Curanderas* do and why people seek their help for both health and personal problems. It further serves as a descriptive guide for professional health care, religious and social-service providers, as well as many individuals who interact with Hispanics in professional settings.

This book is a conglomeration of many different sources and is sorely-needed resource for understanding the cultural realities and health disparities of millions of *Hispanics* in the United States today. This includes thousands of recent immigrants.

Grandma's Remedies and Advice, further seeks to clarify, for health and social care providers, the importance of the role that cultural competencies play in provider interaction with *Hispanic* and other cultural minorities.

It attempts to fill the gap in cultural competencies related to the *Hispanic* population because there isn't anything which is easily available to them in regards to *Curanderismo.* Health and social care providers must understand these aspects of *Hispanic* culture in order to better serve the *Hispanic* community.

This book is an opportunity to experience and study the many assorted cases they encounter in their work with *Hispanics* but never experience with valuable background information.

These cultural perspectives provide a rare opportunity for contextualized mini-cases based on real life experiences.

Additionally, Your *Grandmothers' Guide to Hispanic Remedies &* Advice, provides the reader with a priceless view into the not widely seen or completely understood world of *Curanderismo.* This is especially true in that it provides us with an attempt to understand the mysterious world of *Curanderismo* practicing a unique blend of folk Catholicism and folk healing.

While often misunderstood by religious officials, health-care providers and social service workers, the practice and utilization of *Curanderas,* thrives in the United States and Mexico and throughout Latin America today. The *Hispanic* population, irrespective of socioeconomic level or education, maintains a widespread cultural belief in folk religion and folk medicine.

Wherever *Hispanic* populations are found the number of persons who consult *curanderos,* spiritualists, card readers, herbalists and many other alternative practitioners in the *Hispanic* community grows annually.

Please note that *Curanderismo* never serves as a substitute for the qualified advice and treatment by medical doctors, social care or religious professionals.

However, understanding *Curanderismo,* its beliefs and rituals, provides critical assistance to the interaction between professional caregivers and *Hispanics* in real-life scenarios.

Studies in cultural competency have clearly shown that consultation with *Curanderas,* when practiced alongside modern medicine, social, psychological and religious counseling, bridges the gulf of misunderstanding that exists between these two different, and at times opposing, belief systems.

While numerous religious symbols are introduced and discussed in this book, the book is not about religion nor does it promote religious beliefs or the recommendation of one belief system over another. Religious symbolism is an essential part of *Curanderismo* and is an everyday cultural reality for most Hispanics.

This book abounds with folk remedies and spells prescribed by *Curanderas*; and suggests that we learn and understand them not use them.

This book does not suggest or promote that people in need visit a *Curandera.* What this book does is provide you with the most comprehensive glimpse into present-day *Curanderismo* currently available.

The popularity of *Curanderismo*, in all its aspects, is especially due to the burgeoning *Hispanic* media industry. The events occurring in the United States and Mexico, Puerto Rico or in Columbia today appear on Spanish-language newscasts in the lower Rio Grande Valley of Texas, Chicago, and Los Angeles on the same day.

Hence, the Spanish language is a special culturally bond topic that most *Hispanics* share and the spiritual world is the glue that binds them.

Curanderas practicing their local, site-based, healing arts are now complemented by the availability and anonymity of private consultations. The boundaries of distance, access and culture in consultations are the strongest part of *Curanderismo*. People in need of spiritual help and healing, who would never actually visit a *Curandera* in person, consult them online with impunity. The privacy of Internet use has assisted in increasing the use of *Curandera* consultations especially in times when health care is more difficult to access.

In the United States, medical education has generally failed to meaningfully and systematically incorporate an understanding of cultural competency in its curricula as it relates to *Hispanic* populations. There are, however, acknowledged exceptions and the federal government along with many universities' health-science centers, and health-related organizations have championed the notion of teaching and implementing cultural competencies in recent years.

In spite of all that we have learned about the importance culture plays in the delivery of health care,

Hispanics continue to be one of the least understood ethnic groups in the American health care delivery system.

Each year the American population grows more culturally diverse. We must ask and answer the question, "Should health-care professionals be concerned about mastering cultural competencies related to *Hispanics* in their practice?"

In general, *Hispanic* populations are faced with limited resources and this has exacerbated their need to access alternative and complementary health-care delivery systems at a basal level.

Health-care professionals must construct and accept new and effective health-care models that take culture into consideration in treating *Hispanics* as well as all immigrant populations.

The success of future health-care delivery systems requires that modern medicine and culturally-appropriate alternatives be incorporated into a new functioning paradigm where understanding *Curanderismo* is a key concept.

Modern medicine should take a position of open-mindedness relative to *Curanderas*. Medicine's position should be one of scientific inquiry and not of intolerance. Medical practitioners should be continuously vigilant of patients' beliefs, values and behaviors; seeking knowledge on the cultural issues that shape individual health models.

Cultural beliefs are critical in diagnosing disease, epidemiology, ethnopharmacology, and complementary health practices. Medical and social service providers should develop the communication skills necessary to elicit information from patients and their families as well as to comprehend their personal beliefs.

Information empowers medicine in participatory decision-making regarding health-care delivery. Only when cultural systems and the medical field cooperate will the health-care delivery system be competently able to provide essential health care needed by Hispanics, along with other underserved and/or economically-marginalized populations.

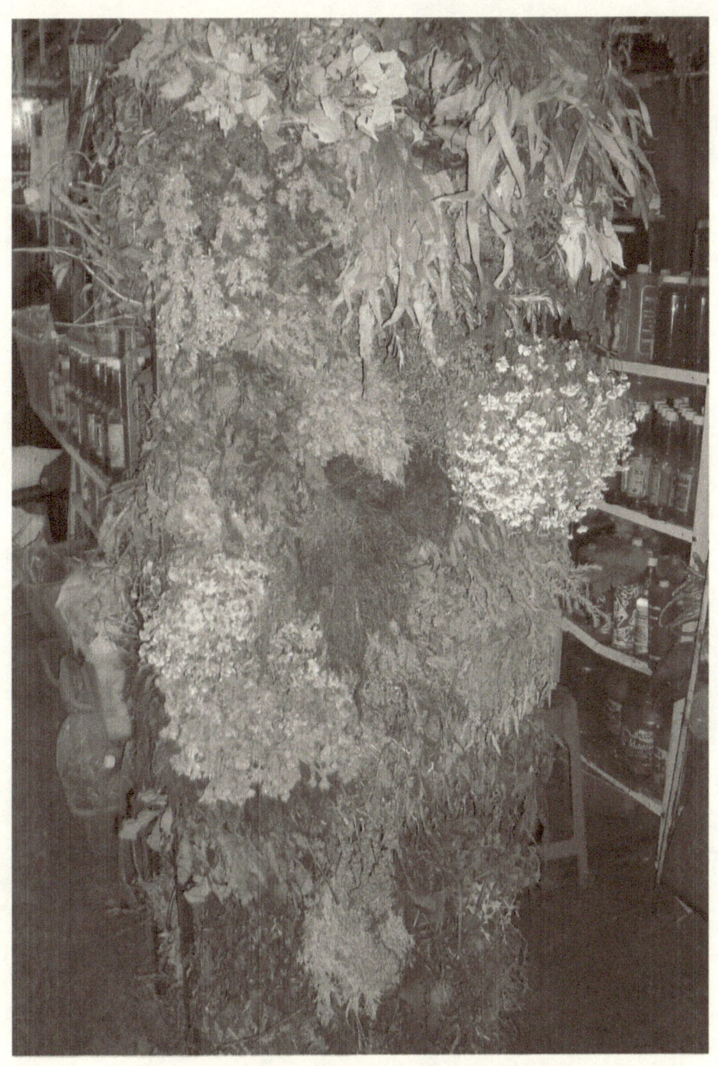

*Fresh medicinal Plants for sale at the
Mercado Sonora In Mexico City*

Part 1
Remedies for Home and Family

BRACERO CAMPFIRE

I first heard about *Curanderas* when I was a young boy in the 1950s. I picked cotton on my grandmother's ranch with migrant farm workers called *braceros* who would tell stories around the campfire at night.

In the 1940s and 1950s the legend of folk saints was in its formative stage and the stories of miraculous cures were being carried northward from Mexico to the border with the United States and then into the American Southwest and Midwest.

The legends of famous *Curanderas* were carried by Mexican migrant farm workers called *braceros* as they migrated northward through the cotton fields, and from citrus orchards to garden patches. Many of the original storytelling *braceros*, were rural farm hands or *campesinos*.

After a long day in the cotton fields, it was not practical to make the long walk back to the farmhouse. I was a 10-year-old son of the ranch owners and lived with the *braceros*. I thank my grandmother for the lessons I learned.

I learned about Mexico's most famous folk healers around a *bracero* campfire just as many others my age. That is exactly how the legends were passed on from generation to generation in those days.

I slept on the ground around the campfires like all of the others. I was just another wide-eyed *bracero* kid, picking cotton under the hot Texas-Mexican sun hoping for September to come, crying out to *Barbas de Oro,* to send the cooling winds indicating that it was time to go back to the comfort of my schoolhouse.

Over the years, I have recounted this story many times, whenever I am asked how I first learned about *Curanderas*.

The women in the field-camp made *tortillas* by hand and cooked up pots of delicious concoctions. There was always plenty of rice, beans and *tortillas*. We worked and sweat all day and ate and slept together in the field-camp at night. I marveled about how respectful the children were as they waited patiently to be fed.

Our fathers, who had toiled all day under the July sun of the *canícula*, the dog days of summer, were always fed first, followed by the children, who were always dutiful. The women would serve themselves last. As they did then, and so today, the women sacrificed themselves to support their hard-working families.

The campfire crackled and reflected ethereal flames on the bronzed faces of the workers, as each evening, one by one, someone would tell a tale, only to be bested by the next story. And so, it went until the last tale was told or everyone had fallen asleep.

I learned about the dog days of summer, called the *canícula*, about *Curanderas* and saints and devils and heard stories about *brujas* or witches and forest elves called *duendes,* who were cousins of Irish Leprechauns. They were said to be all around us all the time.

It was then that I first heard about the mysterious miracle-working, man-child of the desert they called *El Niño Fidencio*. For reasons I do not understand, the folk tales about miracles and healing always fascinated me.

I am often asked how I became interested in anthropology and in *Curanderismo*. I learned from my spiritual path, my personal sojourn, and memories which will endure for my lifetime. This little book will help my memories endure beyond my lifetime. This is just the most recent installment of my path.

FOLK PHARMACY
HIERBERÍA- BOTÁNICA

What is a *hierbería*, also spelled *yerbería?* I have asked my wife several times about her visits to places called *hierberías*. Each time, all she would tell me is that I would not understand. She doesn't want to recognize that I understand more about *Hispanic* culture and folk ways than she knows and that I would like to learn more.

I see some similarities and some differences between these *hierberías* she visits. I also notice that she always goes to these places after she has spoken to her mother or her sister on the phone. In some of these places they have card readers or fortune tellers who read the fortuning telling cards or *La Baraja* for a fee.

Most hierberías have all sorts of remedies. Some stores seem to have all sorts of religious items such as candles and saint's prayer cards. I see these places everywhere we go in *Hispanic* communities, whether they are in Chicago or in the Rio Grande Valley of Texas. These businesses carry all kinds of popular Mexican products.

I see different cultural items such as medallions, candles, oils, perfumes, amulets, talismans, powders, spiritual lotions, potions, some alleged to have divine, magical, mystical, magical power. Some of these products sold at *hierberías* raise many questions in my mind.

In some of these stores I notice that the lady death or *Santísima Muerte* seems to be growing in popularity. I have seen some products that are alleged to do good things and others that seem to be meant to do harm.

Just the other day, we went to this *hierbería* where they had a *Curandera* present in a consulting room. My wife said she needed a ritual cleansing or *limpia* ritual done on her. She and the *Curandera* went into the secluded room in the rear of the store where she says she had a consultation with the Curandera who performed the ritual cleansing.

Historically and traditionally, *hierberías* were places where freshly-picked medicinal and prepared herbs and spices could be purchased.

Curanderas often give their clients a written prescription, or *receta* by the *Curandera* to take to the *hierbería* to be filled. Just like the medical doctor gives us a prescription to take to the pharmacy. All medicinal plants were used in the *Hispanic* home.

Home remedies with the power to heal have been in the market places as trade products since ancient times. The original term in English for the pharmacy is apothecary, and in Spanish, *botica*.

Human cultures have a natural ability to evolve in infinite ways and throughout history has addressed life's ills, adversities, problems, situations and issues.

The herbalist, or *hierbero,* is a specialist in the knowledge of healing herbs. Religion has always been associated with the healing arts and so it is common to find religious items of all faiths and different cultural beliefs for sale in these important folk pharmacies.

Ideologies based on the concept of good and evil as well as the concept of power, both positive and negative, have found their ways into the modern *hierbería*.

Today's *hierberías* started out as small street herb stands and have evolved into major store front businesses.

Additionally, because the *hierbería*, like any other business, is market driven, the items of material culture sold have mixed and combined distinct cultural beliefs. The reason for this is to produce remedies for the human condition with solutions to complex and cross-cultural questions. This consists of persistent and annoying life problems with the hierberías offering spiritual options, and, sometimes, answers and cures.

The indigenous peoples of the world have ancient traditions which identify the use of medicinal plants. The study of medicinal plants is so ancient that the Holy Bible lists approximately 60 plants used for medicines and all play roles in *Hispanic* culture.

Sixteenth-century Catholic priests brought the plants mentioned in the bible to the new world and incorporated them into clerical practice and rituals.

Additionally, all of the esoteric and magical materials that are used by the diverse practices and beliefs of pre-hispanic *Hispanics* are available through *hierberías* and *botánicas*.

In her book, *Pestilence and Headcolds: Encountering Illness in Colonial Mexico*, Fields points out that the concept of the pharmacy, or *botica*, is one that pre-dates the arrival of the Spaniards. The Spanish colonizers licensed and regulated all native pharmacies in 16th century Mexico.

The pharmacist, or *boticario,* held a position of high esteem in the community, and was the *"only establishment that was licensed to sell the public ready-made medicines or have a physician's prescription filled."*

The first Roman Catholic priests in Mexico regarded a certain representation of Mary the mother of God depicted as *Madonna* and *Child* as *Our Lady of Pharmacy.* This representation is believed to have had a Germanic origin.

In colonial Mexico, pharmacists were required to demonstrate a solid knowledge of the medicinal properties of several hundred plants, animals and minerals.

Today's *Curanderas,* retain ancient medical and esoteric knowledge, but on a much smaller scale. The oldest-known Aztec manuscript documenting an herbal in 16th century Mexico lists 251 plants while the Spanish priest Sahagún, who studied folk medicine in colonial Mexico, was able to identify 225 medicinal plants used by the Aztecs. Interestingly, the two lists contain fewer than 20 duplicates placing the total Aztec herbal at close to 500 medicinal plants.

FOLK SAINTS
SANTOS POPULARES

You hear about so many different spirits and folk saints these days. I have trouble keeping them all straight. Who is who and which ones are good or bad? Grandmother, please help me understand all these spirits and entities.

There have always been saints and folk saints in the Catholic Church. There are numerous folk saints such as the *Santo Niño de Atocha, Pedrito Jaramillo, La Santa Muerte and El Niño Fidencio.*

The saints of the church are tried and true and the primary folk saints are also known to be spirits of light. Recently, a whole new group of folk entities and spirits have appeared such as *Jesus Malverde*, that are popular in the media.

The most popular and dangerous folk saint is *La Santísima Muerte*, or Holy Death. Others you see and hear about are *El Niño Fidencio, Jesus Malverde, Juan Soldado, Pancho Villa, Maximón*, various *Indios, gypsies*, and *folk doctors*, and many other popular saints, or *santos populares*.

For example, the *Niño Fidencio* is generally regarded as a good folk saint of healing and basic human needs and is celebrated in March and October each year. My advice to you is not to join a cult, or *culto*, of regional folk saints. Stick to what you know is good and time honored. Pray to the Catholic Church and especially that Catholic priests speak to the importance of understanding and tolerating multicultural beliefs. Santa Mónica, August 27, is often invoked to enlighten Catholics and to bring them back to the Catholic Church. Ask Santa Teresa de Ávila, celebrated on October 15, to fill you with the grace of the Holy Spirit.

Many people in northern Mexico and south Texas have grown up in families where faith in folk saints like *El Niño Fidencio* and faith in the *Virgen de Guadalupe* is strong. Ordinary folks across the countryside assign popular sainthood, or *santificación popular*, to favored local miracle workers, thaumaturge, or *taumaturgos*.

This is perfectly normal since their faith fits into the parallel world of folk religion which is juxtaposed with institutional religion. As such, their faith and devotion to the *Niño* is comparable to Catholic saints and they most often claim to be Catholics. Often, innocent people are surprised to learn that faith in the *Niño Fidencio* is not recognized by the Roman Catholic Church, while he is recognized by the Mexican National Catholic Church founded by Mexican President Plutarco Elias Calles who initiated the Cristero Revolt against the Roman Catholic Church.

Acceptance of spirits and the supernatural is rooted in hundreds of years of tradition by Native American groups in Latin America combined with medieval Catholic beliefs and rituals brought from Europe. In today's practice of *Curanderismo,* the traditions of Native America, Europe and the Americas have been combined and mixed with those from Africa and Asia in what is called religious syncretism.

GRANDMA'S MEDICINE CHEST

Grandmother always helped us with our school projects, especially when they were about her. Now I am working with a team of students and our class project is to re-create a list of household items and substances that the old *Curandera* who lived in our neighborhood and our grandmothers and great-grandmothers used to heal us with when we were ill.

That is, in a time when there were no pharmacies. My part of our project is to construct a list of things that our Mexican and Mexican American mothers used back in the day. Many people, not just *Hispanics,* remember the old *Curandera* home remedies our grandmothers used to use when the family was sick.

The list is lengthy but here are the ones that I still use today that I know were also used in the old days: **vapor** rub; camphor; iodine; merthiolate; mercurochrome; fresh hen's eggs; lemons; alum rock; candles of all kinds; arnica and many other freshly cut herbs from the yard; castor oil; spider web; mineral oil; olive oil; cod liver oil; salt; sugar; fresh honey; laxatives; *piloncillo*; purgative; hot water bottle; soaps; *jabón de barra* or *jabón de la paloma*; *amarillo* or *blanco*; volcanic; *linimento blanco* ; kerosene; rubbing alcohol; *parche Guadalupano*; Ipecac; *cataplasma*; vinegar; chicken soup and broths; aspirin; sulfur; gentian violet; *estropajo*; three roses brilliantine; *agua florida*; lard or *manteca de puerco* or *manteca de coyote*; elixirs; tonics; ash or *ceniza;* incense; tobacco; ammonia; and pine oil for disinfecting.

I am sure there are some I have left out, but this is a basic list. There are many websites where you can look up home remedies from a multitude of diverse cultures. It is remarkable how similar our health needs are, and therefore how familiar our healing traditions are. The majority of these items are used by our Hispanic grandmothers. Also, the many indigenous groups that are represented in the makeup of today's *Hispanic* population all had their favorite local plants, animals and minerals used for healing.

For example, astringents are used to heal wounds, cuts and scrapes, coagulants or coagulantes, and styptics or *estípticos,* and vulnerary or *vulnerarios* for stopping bleeding, and are some of the most common items in the *Curandera's* medicine kit. *Arnica* and all kinds of citrus leaves and blossoms are used to stop bleeding as well.

Germicides or *germicidas,* and disinfectants or *desinfectantes* such as sage and rosemary are also used to prevent or treat infection.

On the other hand, there are many household remedies in grandmother's medicine kit that are useful, such as tonics or *tónicos*, stimulants or *estimulantes* and restoratives or *restaurativos*, for fortifying and strengthen underweight children and the elderly.

Many of our beliefs in *Curanderismo* have been handed down from a "culture of illness-healing" derived from colonial Mexico and are still valid today. This, is one of the principal reasons why *Curanderas* are still necessary. They are used to heal our cultural selves.

Numerous authors have pointed out that native healing traditions in the Americas were, and are, a conglomeration of magic and religion, with a prodigious knowledge base of medicinal plants. In the early days, historians attributed native knowledge of the qualities of food and medicine with European origins, but today most believe that the native populations of Mexico had developed a more comprehensive theory of disease than the fabled world of the Greeks and Romans.

It has been said that "Unlike the mostly worthless Hippocratic and Galenic medicine brought to Mexico by the Spaniards, there was a strong empirical basis to the medical practices of the Nahuatl speakers of central Mexico. It is well known that the invaders trusted the treatment of their wounds to Aztec rather than their own doctors, as the former were far more adept as surgeons and curers"

GIFT OF HEALING
DON DE CURAR

I was raised to tolerate all faiths and beliefs. But now my parents and my brothers and sister have converted to a neighborhood evangelical church and they refuse to understand or accept my Catholic beliefs.

I was raised Catholic and we would go to mass and my mother would sometimes take us with her to see my grandmother who was a healer or *Curandera*.

The *Hispanic* preacher at their church told them that the old cultural ways are demonic and that all *Curanderas* are evil. I just can't believe it's true and I refuse to be changed by this person because I know in my heart that he is wrong. In their church, they have a healing ceremony they call laying-on-of-hands, which to me, is no different than the healing techniques my *Curandera* grandmother uses.

Don't the evangelical and the *Curandera* heal with the same Holy Spirit? Don't they both derive their healing powers from the same God? Help me to understand the difference between what *Curandera* do and what the evangelicals do, if anything?

People just like you ask this question all the time. I firmly believe that both the evangelical ministers and the *Curanderas* use the same gift of the Holy Spirit described in the Holy Bible. The laying-on-of-hands for the purpose of healing is a gift to all people and not exclusive to any one religion.

Your family has been swayed by this new neighborhood church that practices faith healing. I have seen this so many times before because these little churches pop up everywhere like mushrooms after a rain. We must pray for them to be tolerant.

Your family shuns you and condemns you because their new preacher tells them to, and they are trying to please him with blind faith. Eventually, they will understand this is wrong but it may take a while and the relation you have with your family will continue to be strained.

I can assure you that seeing a *Curandera* who gives you support in your cultural beliefs is not evil.

Your parents' laying-on-of-hands and your *Curandera's* healing hands are one and the same. I believe that both derive their healing powers from the Holy Spirit. The two healing traditions are simply different cultural manifestations of the same spiritual power.

Evangelicals demand that you repent your ways in order to save your soul. I believe that their intolerance is what's wrong and that they should respect your beliefs as you respect theirs.

Curanderismo is often condemned as the worshiping of false gods or paganism. In reality, the Holy Bible lists the Seven Gifts of the Holy Spirit, including the gift of healing and condemns the worshiping of false prophets.

The Holy Bible does not speak of religion, so any culturally-based healing practice that calls upon God must be using the same power of the Holy Spirit; it is simply in a different cultural form. It should be noted that authentic *Curanderas* always work with the forces of good against evil.

SPECIALISTS
LOS ESPECIALISTAS

I found the *El Niño Fidencio Curanderismo Research Project* on the Internet and it is just what I have been looking for. I am a Hispanic high-school student and I have chosen to write my senior paper on *Curanderismo* because I am told that long ago my great-grandmother was a *Curandera*.

I have always had this interest in the back of my mind like the spirit of my great-grandmother is urging me to find out about it. One of my aunts even says that I have her "gift." I have found a lot of material on the Internet but could you please help me by explaining how many different kinds of *Curanderas* there are?

There are many different kinds of *Curanderas*. Many are specialists in certain areas just like doctors. For example, the *sobadora*, is a folk massage therapist, and an expert in realigning bundles of nerves and bones just like a chiropractor. Their work can heal tremendous pain throughout the body and affected area. While not generally thought of as a *Curandera*, persons who have the gift and ability to work with their hands are highly valued in a culture which has historically performed physical labor.

The *sobadora* may also have other functions such as bonesetter, or *huesera*. Bone setting is, for all practical purposes, a lost art since emergency room treatment for broken bones is readily available most places.

There are many other specialties in *Curanderismo*. *Hierberas*, or herbalists, are persons who identify the medicinal plants of the countryside, or *campo*, and know of their preparation and use. Specialists in this area gather and dry the plants and, in some cases prepare *compuestos* or herbal mixtures very much like a pharmacist would before the advent of preprepared or patent medicine called *medicina de patente.*

In fact, the folk pharmacy is called the *hierbería* or *botánica.* As in modern pharmacies, *hierberías* now sell a wide variety of items including, but not limited to, fresh herbs. Many medicinal plants used by Hispanics are still very popular and are easily found in neighborhood grocery stores where there is a large *Hispanic* population.

There are lengthy catalogues containing the material sold in *hierberías* or the *materia medica* needed for the modern practice of *Curanderismo.*

The naturalist, or *naturista,* is a modern term for the specialist who practices healing using all natural ingredients and is the modern form of the *hierbera,* or herbal specialist. Naturalists are often found in cities and practice right alongside medical doctors; but they don't identify as *Curanderas.*

Another very important specialist is the midwife or *partera.* Midwifery is an ancient art and one that is highly revered and practiced in Mexico as well as other Latin American countries and throughout the world. For example, in Mexico, *parteras* were trained and licensed long before it was popular in the United States.

This is why unsuspecting women from Mexico often seek midwives or *parteras* in the United States expecting that they have the same training when they often do not.

Other important subdivisions of *Curanderismo* include healers who only work with physical or material items; they are said to work *materialmente*. They include, for example, the *hierbera, sobadora* and *partera* who work with their folk knowledge and with physical items like creams, salves, and oils using their hands.

There are, however, *Curanderas* who work on a higher plane, or with their minds, these are often called *mentalistas* or mentalists.

Mentalistas will concentrate their gaze on an object like a crystal ball; bowl of clear water or a religious icon and in their concentrated state of consciousness will look or "see" into the life of a questioner. Often, they seem to be in a trance and are silent for a time; they "return" to consciousness with an answer or with a recommendation from the spirit world.

Ocultista is another term and form of *Curanderismo.* Like the naturalist, *ocultista* is a modern term for a person who practices the hidden or esoteric arts, hence the use of the term occult or unseen. The different terms vary from region to region and from city to countryside.

Curanderas never think of themselves as *ocultistas,* although in the cities the term is not uncommon.

Another practice of *Curanderas* is to work spiritually, and, hence, the term *espiritista*.

The *espiritista* is actually a trance medium who, while in a trance state, works with or brings down a spirit. The medium channels the spirit of a once-living entity which speaks and acts through the medium to bring about the healing through consultation with the spirit.

The term shaman is also well known and is used to refer to a native or indigenous healer. All shamans are healers, but not all healers are shamans.

Shamanism is often associated with altered realities and supernatural states of consciousness. Basically, shamanism and *Curanderismo* have very similar practices. Shamanism is a term adopted by anthropologists to describe medicine men and women in Native American and other populations. Both shamanism and *Curanderismo* incorporate the material culture and the spirituality of native beliefs. It doesn't matter where the native people or cultures come from. Shamanistic beliefs are universal in the human population. I have been very fortunate to have met and work with many shamans who have adopted me as a student. They are from many diverse North and Meso-American cultures during my lengthy career.

There is basically no difference in the two terms and the practices of one are common to the practices and beliefs of the other. One of my closest teachers was a Huichol shaman elder I met from the Mexican state of Jalisco. I met him on a spiritual journey to *Real de Catorce* in the Mexican state of *San Luis Potosí* about 30 years ago. He adopted me as his student and has taught me quite a lot, including the art of the *temazcal* sweat lodge, and how to conduct a *peyote-mitote*. Both are healing and cleansing rituals. Another was a Cherokee shaman or medicine man.

In Latin American culture, the card reader is a very important category of folk practitioner. A card reader is said to throw the cards or the *baraja*, usually they use the Spanish tarot deck. There are many different styles of card spreads and traditions which date back a thousand years. The more modern card readers are usually found in urban areas and may use the European tarot deck like the well-known, *Rider-Waite* deck while the more traditional card readers in the *Hispanic* community almost always use the *Spanish tarot deck.*

This form of divination called cartomancy, or card reading, continues to be extremely popular and pervasive in the Latin community today. Most card readers do not think of themselves as *Curanderas,* while some may actually operate in both realms.

Just as there is a God and a devil, just as there is good and evil, there are persons who practice both good and evil traditions. Generally speaking, we think of *Curanderas* as persons who aid their communities and who therefore do "good."

Curanderas, generally work in one of the traditions at a time. Good is said to be performed by using the right hand. However, there are those who are dedicated to the traditions and forces of evil and some are said to work with the left hand, and are considered sinister. Some work with both sides, good and evil. When this occurs, they usually keep these practices separate from one another. They operate in different spaces and places, on different days and at different hours of practice. Witchcraft must always be kept separate and cannot be mixed with good healing.

In every *Hispanic* community, both practitioners of good and evil exist and are often active against each other; carrying on wars of the witches, *Curanderas* vs. *brujas,* healers vs. witches, for decades.

We call the people who practice witchcraft and whose job is to harm people or to make them sick, *brujas* or warlocks or witches.

Brujas, or witches, fall into many categories. *Brujas* may use completely indigenous traditions gleaned from active native groups in Mexico or other places. Or they may use traditions that have been popularized by mixing the ancient with the modern and the Eastern with the Western traditions.

Active today, are many varieties of cults which have grown out of these traditions including satanic cults or devil-worshiping cults such as the ones with their origin in *Catemaco, Veracruz,* considered the home of witchcraft in Mexico. While cults are not a familiar part of *Hispanic* culture, recently notable subcultures have sprung up surrounding both real and imagined folk figures.

Most notable is the recent popularity of *La Santísima Muerte* in *Hispanic* culture. Sub-cultures and cults are generally regionalized and surround a popular folk figure, such as *Malverde, Pancho Villa, Juan Soldado, El Niño Fidencio* and many others.

Curandera specialists no longer commonly include the tooth puller, or *sacamuelas,* the person who specialized in sucking out illnesses, or *soplador;* the enlightened healer or *alumbrada*; the *algebrista/huesero,* bonesetter; the sangradora or bleeder; and the person who prayed illness away or *ensalmador.* All of these specializations are included in today's common term of *Curandera.*

From where do *Curanderismo* and popular religions emanate? In his book, *The Church in the Barrio,* Roberto Treviño states in speaking about the origin of what he calls "ethno-religion," and quotes from the work of Roberto Goizueta,

"The Mexican Americans in Texas and in the Southwest carried on this ethno-religion that, in the spirit of its

medieval and Indian roots, made room for faith healing and other practices deemed superstitious by clergy; favored saint veneration, home altar worship, and community-centered religious celebration that blurred the line between the sacred and the secular. These are all important practices of Curanderismo. Ethno-religious rites tended to simultaneously and selectively participate in institutional Catholic Church practices, yet hold the Church at arm's length. Ethno Catholicism was essentially countercultural, as it represented an organic, holistic worldview…at odds with post-Enlightenment notions of time and space, of the material and the spiritual, and of the person's place within time and space, within the material and spiritual dimensions of reality."

The first Europeans in Mexico encountered a culture that was a syncretic or mixture of medical and religious beliefs that has passed down to *Curanderismo. Curanderas* of today's America are not only lost in space and time; they are the agents of its interpretation. The male healer is the *curandero* and the female healer is the *Curandera.*

Curanderismo is a term coined by researchers and those who study *curanderos/as.* It refers to the practice or the art of folk healing in the *Hispanic* community. The *Curandera's* response outlines the many specializations and practices that are ordinarily categorized under the title of *Curanderismo.* There is a new generation of *Hispanics* and others, who want and need to know about the world of the *Curandera.*

Ancient and modern books have documented through literature and votive paintings that the stock in trade of *Curanderas* has changed only slightly since the arrival of Europeans in Latin America. Each *Curandera* has his or her spiritual tool kit or *herramienta espiritual.*

In her book, *Pestilence and Headcolds: Encountering Illness in Colonial Mexico*, Sherry Fields states, *"This is the world of the sick-room, both a physical space abounding with strange tonics and brews, bleedings and leeches, Curanderas and barber-surgeons, and saints and virgins, as well as a cultural space complete with its own structures of meaning."* Today, little has changed in the healing room of the *Curanderas* of the borderlands.

In Mexico, as everywhere else, there were always those who practiced the healing arts outside of the law. In colonial Mexico they were called intruders or *intrusos*. To an extent, this still exists today with many persons pretending to practice *Curanderismo* while knowing little or nothing about it.

There have always been folk saints like *Pedrito Jaramillo, Santo Niño de Atocha and El Niño Fidencio*. The saints of the church are tried and true and the primary folk saints are also known to be spirits of light. Recently, a whole new group of folk entities and spirits have appeared, that are popular in the media and at *hierberías*.

Today, the most popular and dangerous folk saint is *La Santísima Muerte*, or Holy Death. Some others you see and hear about are *Malverde, Juan Soldado, Pancho Villa, Maximón*, and many others who are regarded as popular saints, or *santos populares*.

My advice to you is not to get caught up in the cult, or *culto*, of regional folk saints and stick to what you know is good and time honored. Pray to Saint John Mary Vianney, August 4, that the Catholic Church and especially Catholic priests open their minds to the importance of understanding and tolerating multicultural beliefs.

Many people in northern Mexico and south Texas have grown up in families with faith and devotion in folk saints like the Virgen de Guadalupe. Ordinary folks across the countryside assign popular sainthood, or *santificación popular*, to favored miracle workers thaumaturges, or *taumaturgos*.

This is perfectly normal since their faith fits into the parallel world of folk religion which is juxtaposed with institutional religion. As such, their faith and devotion are comparable to Catholic saints and often claim to be Catholics.

Acceptance of spirits and the supernatural is rooted in hundreds of years of tradition by Native American groups in Latin America combined with medieval Catholic beliefs and rituals brought from Europe. In today's practice of *Curanderismo,* the traditions of Europe and the Americas have been combined and mixed with those from Africa and Asia in people's beliefs but not sanctioned by the Catholic Church.

Year in and year out, the religious seasons and holidays, celebrate saints' days and other special days with common prayers, practices and rituals by both the Catholic Church and *Curanderas.* Regardless if the saint is in the church or in the home of the *Curandera*, the practices are the same. This fact unites the two traditions in the minds of the faithful.

Guerra states that, *"Saints were patrons of various diseases, illness frequently took on moral tones, and remedical books customarily included enormous numbers of prayers, novenas, and religious tracts for preventing and curing disease"*

While not all *Curanderas* follow the traditional santoral or church liturgical calendar today, it is coming back into favor by the younger generation which wants to do things the way their grandparents did.

Through the centuries many of the Catholic saints have developed traditions, rituals and cult followings including their celebrations at certain times of the year. In her book, Fields states:

"In January 1737, procesiones and novenarios to various divine images were made through the streets of Mexico City. To ask for relief from the fiery epidemic that people are suffering from in this kingdom. The Mexican cult of saints has origins in the pilgrimage traditions practiced in medieval Europe." The same traditions practiced in colonial Mexico are practiced by our *Curanderas* today.

HOME REMEDIES
REMEDIOS CASEROS

Many people, not just *Hispanics*, remember the old *Curandera* home remedies our grandmothers used when the family was sick. The list is lengthy but here are the ones that I still use today that I know were also used in the old days they include but are not limited to the following:

Vapor rub; camphor; iodine; merthiolate; mercurochrome; fresh hen's eggs; lemons; alum rock; candles of all kinds; freshly cut herbs from the yard; castor oil; spider web; mineral oil; olive oil; cod l liver oil; salt; sugar; fresh honey; laxatives; piloncillo; purgative; hot water bottle; soaps; jabón de barra or jabón de la paloma; amarillo or blanco; volcanic; linimento blanco ; kerosene; rubbing alcohol; parche Guadalupano; Ipecac; cataplasma; vinegar; chicken soup and broths; aspirin; sulfur; gentian violet; estropajo; three roses brilliantine; agua florida; lard or manteca de puerco or manteca de coyote; elixirs; tonics; ash or ceniza; incense; tobacco; ammonia; and pine oil for disinfecting. I am sure there are some I have left out, but this is a basic list.

There are many websites where you can look up home remedies from a multitude of diverse cultures such as European, Afro-Caribbean, and Native American. It is remarkable how similar our health needs are, and therefore how similar our healing traditions are.

Grandma always knew how to settle an upset stomach. The *Curandera* has listed the majority of those items that are used by our Hispanic grandmothers. Also, the many indigenous groups that are represented in today's *Hispanic* population all had their favorite local regional plants, animals and minerals used for healing.

For example, astringents are used to heal wounds, cuts and scrapes, coagulants or *coagulantes*, and styptics or *estípticos*, and vulnerary or *vulnerarios* for stopping bleeding. These are some of the most common items in the *Curandera's* medicine kit. *Arnica* and all kinds of citrus leaves and blossoms are used for this purpose as well.

Germicides or *germicidas,* and disinfectants or *desinfectantes* such as sage and rosemary are also used to prevent or treat infection.

On the other hand, there are many household remedies in grandmother's medicine kit that are useful, such as tonics or *tónicos*, stimulants or *estimulantes* and restoratives or *restaurativos*, for fortifying and to strengthen underweight children and the elderly.

Many of our beliefs in *Curanderismo* have been handed down to us from a "culture of healing" derived from colonial Mexico and are still valid today. This is one of the principal reasons why *Curanderas* are still necessary. They heal our cultural selves.

Numerous authors have pointed out that native-healing traditions in the Americas were, and are, a conglomeration of magic and religion, with a prodigious knowledge base of medicinal plants.

In the early days, historians attributed native knowledge of the "qualities" of food and medicine with European origins, but today most believe that the native populations of Mexico had developed a more comprehensive theory of disease than the fabled world of the Greeks and Romans. Coe and Whittaker point out that:

"Unlike the mostly worthless Hippocratic and Galenic medicine brought to Mexico by the Spaniards, there was a strong empirical basis to the medical practices of the Nahuatl speakers of central Mexico. It is well known that the (Spanish) invaders trusted the treatment of their wounds to Aztec rather than their own doctors, as the former were far more adept as surgeons and curers"

MY PILGRIMAGE
PEREGRINACIÓN PERSONAL

I was born with a birth defect, and while it was not life threatening, it did have the potential to cause a lifelong disability if not corrected. My father and mother who were both Marines had little recourse and places to turn for help in the post-war years. My father's mother, my grandmother, *Concepcion* or *Conchita* asked her son to pray to the *Virgen de Guadalupe*, to ask her to intercede with her Son, Our Lord, asking for no less than a miracle for their baby boy.

The miracle was granted, my experimental surgery was performed at the University of California at Los Angeles Medical Center in 1947. There was no charge for the young Marine Corps family.

A couple of years later, my grandmother reminded her son not to forget the promise that he had made to the *Virgen* and that he was obliged to complete his promise or *manda* by making a pilgrimage to her holy site.

The miracle that was granted required my father to take his family on a pilgrimage to a shrine in Mexico in order to fulfill his *manda*, or spiritual burden, and promise he made to the *Virgen*.

It's now half a century later and I am 50 years old. My father and mother had never told me the story of my surgery, the miracle received or our pilgrimage to give thanks. Thus, as a middle-aged man, I began having dreams and flashbacks of the trip we took to Mexico when I was only three years old.

Wanting to know more about this aspect of my life and an explanation for my lifelong devotion to the *Virgen de Guadalupe*, I asked my aging and sickly father to tell me about it.

It was only then that the fantastic story was told to me for the very first time. My elderly father could remember only generalities, but not exactly where the place was that he took his young family and son.

I wanted to return there and to take my father back there before his death in an effort to repay my father for the faith he had so many years ago, and for asking the *Virgen* for my miracle.

I asked the *Virgen de Guadalupe* through a *materia*, or trance medium, for directions. As a Mexico traveler, I was very familiar with Mexican highways.

The *Virgen de Guadalupe* told me spiritually that she was familiar with my case and instantly revealed the pilgrimage location as *El Chorrito* in the northern Mexican state of *Tamaulipas*. Plans were begun to take my father and my *materia* on a pilgrimage to *El Chorrito*.

The *Virgen* through my trance-medium of *El Niño Fidencio*, told me that she had been waiting all these years for me to discover my story and that I should take my father there as soon as possible. So, within a couple of weeks, my father, my *materia*, her *guardia* and I, made the trek southward from the Texas border to *El Chorrito*, a day trip of about 200 miles.

We set off early in the morning and had so much joy that day, as we visited there half a century later, and thanked the *Virgen* for my miracle. Not long after that, my father died, but before his death, we were able to close the circle on the most important spiritual connection a father and son can have: love.

This beautiful story points out the connection between Our Lady of Guadalupe and her helpers in heaven including all of the Saints. This story is particularly touching for several reasons.

The *Virgen* helped me to remember this important event in my life. She uses one of her *materias* on earth to help me and I am able to take my father there thanking the *Virgen de Guadalupe* for the miracle I received in my life and explains my lifelong devotion to her.

I am aware of countless stories of people who have a devotion to a certain saint or *Virgen* and was not sure why. Like you, some find out why, but in most cases they never do. I was lucky. Nevertheless, they do know that their devotion is real and profound.

Hispanic culture is one of faith and deep devotion. *Hispanics* revere the many aspects of the *Virgen* and the saints who serve as their spiritual protectors; helping them to cope with life's many dilemmas.

This book shares many of those. Devotion to the *Virgen* of *Guadalupe* for example, is passed on generationally, as exemplified by this beautiful and heart-rending story.

Hopefully, many others will take their children back along the same path to pilgrimage that began with his grandmother and his ancestors. Most *Hispanics* do not make a distinction between the Catholic Church and folk saints. However, both are equally valid and important in our lives.

GOOD MEDICINE
LA BUENA MEDICINA

I have been the beneficiary of many of my grandma's home remedies and I won't ever forget how she insisted we shake out our shoes every morning before we put them on, to get rid of any scorpions or spiders that might have crawled inside. Sometimes one of us grand kids would scream and the scorpion would run across the floor until an older grandchild, with shoes on, would step on it. Once this happened, you were a believer in grandma's remedies.

When we all went walking in the *monte,* or countryside, with my grandma, we felt safe. She always had a *rebozo,* or shawl tied over her shoulder with some fruit for us and her magical remedies if we needed them.

When one of my cousins scraped against a *maguey* cactus, grandma was ready.

The *maguey* cactus looks like a century plant or *yucca* plant with thick leaves, but has dry pointed leaves that can deeply scratch the fragile flesh of a youngster. It is pretty bad for an adult as well.

My cousin fell into a *maguey* when I was young and I remember what my grandma did for her. Grandma pulled out her pocket knife and sliced a lime, we had picked, in half and squeezed its juice onto the scratch then she massaged the whole area with the half of lime to keep the *maguey* poison from making her arm swell up.

In the *campo* the small rainbow cactus was covered with fine spines and easy to miss while walking but grandma was always ready. One of my cousins tripped, fell into a tiny bunch of rainbow cacti, the result was an armful of the tiny blonde needles that reflect the light spectrum and gives the little barrel-like plants the name of rainbow cactus.

My grandma whipped out one of the braids of hair that comprised her bun and rubbed her loose hair in a circular motion on my cousin's arm until all the tiny spines disappeared. We thought it was magic!

The truth is that the rainbow spines are too fragile to be removed by tweezers and human hair will pull them out of skin and then brushed out of the hair. Since they are not as thick as a human hair, there is something about human hair that grabs them when they come in contact with the hair shaft being rubbed against the spine-filled skin.

I have forgotten a lot of remedies I once knew. If we were stung by a bee or wasp in the *campo,* or countryside, grandma would put a cup in our hands and tell us to go pee in it while she used the pocket knife like an old-fashioned straight razor and lay the blade almost flat against the skin, scraping the stinger out. Then she would pour the urine on the sting neutralizing the poison.

Most people don't know that urine is sterile for the first minutes after it is expelled and grandma always rubbed it off and patted the area with a cloth that was doused with *pulque,* a homemade tequila-like brew that she had in a tiny bottle; carried in her *rebozo,* along with her many bandaging rags. She never left her house without her medicine bag.

HEALING GARDEN
JARDÍN DE CURACIÓN

Grandma, I'm writing to you because I was remembering my great aunt and how she raised me after my mother passed away. You had given me several ways to protect my house, and a braided garlic hanging next to the doors going outside brought back many wonderful memories.

My great aunt had a wonderful green thumb and the adobe wall that surrounded the house was filled with old juice and vegetable cans that were nailed onto the wall. My auntie made small holes in the can bottoms and filled them with dirt. She rooted geraniums, started seedlings, and grew kitchen herbs.

One whole side of her house was planted with corn and elephant garlic, at least that is what she called it. I think others might say it was *ajo macho*, or male garlic, because it was the biggest head of garlic cloves and it had very tall green straight leaves like green onions or scallions. Anyway, it looked really huge to me as a young boy and I loved watering the corn and garlic as much as the bounty of flowers because their bright colors made me happy.

Once a year we would pick the garlic and she would make big four-foot-long braids and she would have me pick red, hot pink and white geraniums, lavender and purple petunias, as well as yellow, orange and red zinnias.

All the beautiful colored flowers would be woven into the garlic wreath and hung to dry under the *enramada*, or shade arbor, so as the flowers dried, they would retain their bright colors and the green garlic stems would turn as gold as dried wheat.

When the garlic strands were ready, we would say a prayer as we tied red satin ribbons into bows on each end. The prayer was a blessing for our home, but I don't remember it being the same each time because I was allowed to add my own little prayer at the end of auntie's prayer.

At night, after supper, we would build a fire inside a 55-gallon drum at the back of the lot where a gate prevented our goats and chickens from entering grandma's garden. It was our trash-burning barrel made of metal. Auntie would stand up on a kitchen chair and pull the garlic strands from the previous year down from above the front and back doors to the house. Then, she would put them in the fire, watching them burn until they were ash.

Only then, would we hang the new blessed garlic and flower strands above the front and back doors on the four large nails that made them rest on an arch above the doorway.

Auntie explained to me that the old strands had protected our home for a year and were laid to rest. Since they had done their job well, it was time for a new generation of garlic and flowers to take their turn.

I wanted to know why she always insisted that the garlic in the kitchen never be braided and why she called it eating garlic that was kept in a covered ceramic pot with air holes on the side and was never to be placed near the kitchen window.

When garlic strands are for protection, they absorb negativity and jealousy inside or outside the home. That is their purpose. Braiding garlic was an ancient tradition. Auntie would do this to make the strands ornamental because no one would take them apart to use a clove or two for cooking. The ugly thoughts or feelings of others are absorbed into the garlic strands and, if eaten, can make one very sick, especially if the family is a target of other people's envy or witchcraft.

Grandma responded; your auntie was right. They must be replaced once a year and burned. I suspect that the garlic and floral braid was placed in an arch to resemble a church door and her connection to the archangels. As far as the eating garlic goes, it will dry out the juicy cloves if it gets too hot in the sun and rot if it gets too moist. Most garlic pots sold in stores have vents on the sides so that the garlic will not mold in moist, humid or rainy climates.

I hope that this has given you as many fond memories as it has given me an enduring pleasure. Culture is rich and alive in our lives and we must never forget who we are, where we come from and who our ancestors were. After all, they are constantly keeping vigilance over us, fully expecting us to do the right thing.

Hopefully, this little book has stimulated remembrances of your grandmother and family remedies you may have marveled at, wondered about and maybe even forgotten through the years.

Treasure this little book. In the future, it may be the only place you will find this information consolidated into one source. Pass it along to your children. Consider it your personal spiritual-and-cultural reference book handed down to you from your grandmothers and her ancestors.

Grandma was very wise indeed. Most of our grandmothers always kept aloe vera plants in the four corners of their yard as well as in their kitchen where meals were prepared.

I remember that my grandmother put raw onion and parsley into a blender and then strained the juice with cheesecloth and she would have us drink it when we started getting head colds or lung congestions. She also used the pulp for other remedies. Drinking raw onion juice is an ancient and effective remedy for a head cold.

Another household remedy comes from the *mesquite* tree which many thorns that can easily puncture the skin even if the person is wearing leather gloves or chaps if they are on horseback. The *mesquite* thorn must be removed or it can cause blood poisoning and sometimes gangrene.

The poultice my family used for the sores where the *mesquite* thorns were removed was the pulp from the onion and parsley mixed together with garlic and mustard seed mashed in a mortar and pestle then spread on the sore and bandaged. People would change the poultice regularly depending on how long the *mesquite* thorn had been in the skin and whether fever, delirium, and/or blood poisoning was present. Insert three headless needles into the onion or garlic head and place it in Holy Water, do this every day for seven days and then bury the onion or garlic away from your home.

As for the *aloe vera* plant in the kitchen, the gel inside the leaves is commonly used for kitchen burns and the juice can heal scratches or kitchen cuts as well as calming stomachs that have frequent heartburn.

Almost everyone has cherished childhood memories which are especially sweet when they involve remembering and learning under the direction of a grandmother or grandfather along with our many cousins.

Here, we find wonderful memories of grandmother's remedies in a much simpler time. Memories from a time of innocence provide us with the framework for our sense of being, for our cultural realities and for our values.

The reality is that most of our grandmother's remedies can be verified as effective when compared to the "official" recipe book of the American Pharmaceutical Association of the early 20th century.

For example, medicated-nasal drops, whether mixed at home or at the corner pharmacy, consisted of oil of eucalyptus, oil of dwarf pine needles and menthol mixed in a light petrolatum liquid. This mixture is still mixed up and used by *Curanderas* today.

As we walk through life, sometimes we encounter a familiar scenario, a particular aroma or hear a sound or voice that stirs a long-forgotten memory. Savor that moment! Your ancestors are conveying a special message to you. Thank You Jamie.

POLTICE
CATAPLASMA

The cataplasma or medicinal patch, *parche*, is an age-old medicinal treatment known from both the old world and the new. Healers placed their favorite healing plant in the concoction placed on the patch. The patch was then placed on ailing or injured part of the body. Grandmother would always prepare a parche for her injured or ailing sons. The patch is hot and an inflammatory usually applied to the back or any other part of the injured body where a strain or sprain has occurred. Since the 19th century the cataplasma has been pre-prepared and available in pharmacies and *Boticas*. This remarkably effective patch is porous and contains heating capsicum. My father who worked with heavy equipment would often send me to the corner store for El Parche Guadalupano.

COLDS AND FLUS
LA GRIPA Y RESFRIADOS

There are hundreds of home remedies for treating the symptoms of colds and the flu, that we call *la gripa* in Spanish. I will share with you just a couple of remedies to put you on the right road. Most stuffy little noses can be helped by rubbing Vicks® below the nostrils and on the child's chest. This is one of the time-tested and favorite *Hispanic* remedies. At night, vaporizers can also help children to breathe and sleep through the night.

For fevers, grandmother prepares a tea made of *sauz*, the willow tree, or *borraja*, the herb borage, or *cardo santo*, blessed thistle, or *epazote de zorrillo*, called wormseed, all heal or *valeriana*, castor bean or *higuerilla*, pennyroyal or marigold or *calendula, caña fistula*, ginger or *jengibre, honeysuckle* or *muicle*, and many others.

All will reduce fever and it would depend on the degree of severity and what is available. See which one works best for your child. At the *hierbería*, there are prepared herbal mixtures called *compuestos* which are ready to use to reduce fever find which one works best for you.

For sore throats and persistent cough, give teas prepared with lemon, onion, garlic, cloves, eucalyptus and honey. Medicinal plants you can give for cough and sore throats also include bay leaves or *laurel*, borage or *borraja*, clematis or *barba de chivo*, marigold or *calendula*, mallow or *malva*, mulberry or *mora*, pomegranate or *granada*, elm or *olmo*, and sumac or *zumaque*. If an upset stomach is part of the problem, prepare a tea made from *manzanilla* or chamomile.

Breathing and respiratory problems and congestion have dozens of remedies that can be used including lavender, *lavándula*, borage, or *borraja*, mustard seed, licorice root, agrimony, *arbol de la cera* or bay berry, bay leaves or *laurel*, sour orange tree leaves, called *naranja agria*, bold or *boldo*, camphor weed or *arnica Mexicana*, common juniper or *enebro*, cudweed or pennyroyal or *poleo*, and many more that are available depending on your location.

You could even start your own home medicinal plant herb garden. For example, basil, mint, rosemary and many other common medicinal plants are available year-round and can be used in teas. Rosemary, or *romero,* works well with chronic coughs.

Always prepare a chicken soup for your sick kids, and keep a record of the remedies that work for you, and you will have your grandmother's medicine chest right there in your home and she will look down upon you lovingly.

STOMACH ACHES
EMPACHO, CÓLICO, Y LATIDO

Grandmother always uses herbs for a "blocked" or upset stomachs or when a child is *empachado* or has *empacho.*

Some children have chronic stomach problems, diarrhea, and vomiting. Everything they eat disagrees with them.

You may need to take your child to the doctor if he does not respond, but it might just be a bad case of *cólico,* or colic. For *cólico,* the best remedy is *té de manzanilla,* or chamomile tea. You could also give him a tea made from *hierbanís,* or anise, or *epazote de zorillo,* or wormseed. Since the child might have an intestinal obstruction called *empacho,* give the child a teaspoon of olive oil with a pinch of salt on the tongue. Grandmother sees all kinds of digestive disorders and there are numerous home remedies for them.

For example, you could take any of the following: agrimony or *agrimonia,* almond or *almendra,* aloe vera or *sávila,* wormseed or *epazote,* anise or *anis,* bay leaf or laurel, bitter wood or *cassia,* black cumin or comino *negro,* blessed thistle or cardo *santo,* mint or *poleo,* cinnamon or *canela,* giant hyssop or *toronjil,* horehound or marrubio, *limón* or *lima*, Mormon tea or *popotillo* and numerous others.

Rub the child's abdomen gently with olive oil for three minutes. Turn the child on his stomach and rub olive oil on his lower back for about three minutes. Place a towel on the lower back and gently pinch the skin using both hands, side by side, using the towel to pull outward until the skin pops.

Repeat this procedure moving lower down the back each time. Pulling and popping the skin on the lower back of the body is the action that causes the *empacho,* or intestinal obstruction, to successfully be dislodged from the intestinal tract, and the digestive system will then begin to function properly. *Empacho* is a term used to describe a condition resulting from an intestinal obstruction caused by a clump of undigested food lodged somewhere within the digestive system. This stomach condition is due to something that the person ate which remained in the intestinal tract or by something consumed that was spoiled.

Contamination of the food or rejection of the food usually occurs because it wasn't sufficiently cooked or was spoiled. This ailment, which is very common in children, can occur in adults as well. All types of stomach and intestinal problems were frequently treated by grandmother with an enema, or *purga.*

Most Hispanics raised in traditional households are familiar with the preventative *purga.* There are many herbal products such as flax seed that serve as antidysentery; antispasmodics such as *calamus* or sweet flag, or yarrow; emetics to induce vomiting and nausea like, *las habas de San Ignacio*; called *purgantes,* or purgatives, and/or herbal laxatives such as Epsom salts and many others.

Cólico and latido are familiar stomach and intestinal problems that *Curanderas* are asked to treat. Simply speaking, colic translates as stomach gas commonly called indigestion. *Latido* literally means throbbing, but also refers to the symptom of nausea.

Because stomach and intestinal problems are so much a part of our human condition, there are literally hundreds of remedies for them which have been passed on generationally.

Grandmother, I know that you were told that I have a *malpuesto* or *brujería,* or witchcraft that caused my problem, but your accident came naturally and not by witchcraft.

I think that the problem is from an old scare or *susto pasado.* It is possible that you can be relieved significantly of your pain.

The cure you need is for *susto,* or a past *susto,* a trauma, fright or pain.

Boil *sávila* and lemon grass together and drink one cup of tea in the morning and another at night for 40 consecutive days. General aches and pains are among the most common physical ailments treated and there are a wide variety of medicinal plants or *plantas medicinales* that can be used.

The plants can be taken as teas, or prepared as saves or ointments and rubbed on the body part that hurts. Some of the most commonly used are, aloe vera or *sávila,* ambrosia or *hierba amarga,* angels trumpet or *florifundo,* black mustard, or *mostaza negra,* boneset or *eupatorium, burro* bush or *hierba del burro, camphor* or *alcanfor, camphor* weed sometimes called *arnica,* Indian plantain or *matarique,* and finally, *nutmeg* or *nuez moscada.*

Commonly, grandmother asks people to eat one garlic capsule and two aloe vera capsules, in the morning and at night, for 40 straight days.

In the Hispanic healing community, there are specialists called bonesetters, or *hueseros,* and massage therapists recognized as *sobadoras.* These folk-specialists often have the uncanny ability to redirect and sort out nerve bundles and to soothe strained muscles. They should always be used to reinforce or complement medical advice.

Often, back problems and bone and joint complications are caused by inflammation. Anti-inflammatory and antispasmodic or *antiespasmódico* and *linimento,* or liniment, such as *volcanico* and *arnica,* are prescribed by grandmother to reduce inflammation.

Kidneywood or *palo azul* is one of the best-known *hierbas* used for reducing swelling. Lemon grass, or *zacate de limón,* is taken as a tea and used to reoxidize the blood. An agent which reintroduced oxygen to the blood is called an antioxidant or in Spanish, *antioxidante.* A common antispasmodic is yarrow, or *milenrama.*

FRIGHT SICKNESS
EL SUSTO

Susto is one of the most common Hispanic folk illnesses. Cut a lemon in half, then rub, squeezing the juice on your knees. Do this for five minutes. Afterward, rub the knees with egg white until the egg white becomes dry and sticky. Leave the egg white on and do not wash it off until your next bath. Prepare a tea made from *salvia* and zacate *de limón.*

In order to cure a child's fright sickness, *susto*, sweep the child with a *piedra alumbre,* or alum rock which you can buy at any *hierbería* or Mexican products store. Use this same rock to do the sweeping, or *barrida.* Set the rock aside each day in a safe place and do not allow anyone to touch it because her *susto* could easily jump to a nearby innocent person.

Dissolve the Alum Rock or *Piedra Alumbre* in water and add either Holy Water or *Siete Machos* lotion to the water. Wash the doors and windows of your home with this mixture. Also protect your Holy objects by rinsing them in Piedra Alumbre water.

You may also find the Piedra Alumbre effective in ridding bad energies from your home. Place the rock in some water with lemon drops and Siete Machos and store the liquid for one month.

Give the child a cup of spearmint, *hierba buena*, basil tea for the same nine days you sweep her. After the ninth day of sweeping, start a fire and burn the alum rock on the hot coals. This will cure the child of *susto.*

Susto is one of the most recurring folk illnesses and may be treated by sweeping alum rock known as *piedra alumbre* over the body of the child or person who is scared, or *asustada.* Usually, this ritual sweeping is repeated for three to nine days in a row.

A person will recognize that they or their loved one was scared or startled. The scare triggers the usual symptoms of fever and sleeplessness. If nausea accompanies the fright sickness, grandmother often advises that an antiemetic herb, *antiémetico*, such as wormseed, against throwing up be given.

Say the Apostles' Creed, or *Credo*, while doing the ritual sweeping. At the end of the ritual, the alum rock must be burned outside the home over hot coals. Many believe that they can see the evil burned into the stone. It's also believed that the image of the person or entity which caused the initial *susto* or soul loss can be reflected in the alum rock.

Severe cases of *susto* or fright sickness are called *desasombro* and can occur in both the waking and sleeping states. This severe case of fright is believed to cause the patient a fever, loss of sleep, desperation and should be treated immediately. There are believed to be even more severe cases of *susto* called, *susto pasado* or *susto meco*.

FALLEN FONTANEL
MOLLERA CAÍDA

Grandmother my mother says my baby may have *mollera caída*, also commonly called *caída de la mollera*. My baby is 10 months old and has been crying day and night for about a week and does not stop being irritable. The doctor checked her out and wants to see her again tomorrow to give us the results of the tests she did on her. Could it be true what my mother says, that my little girl could have *caída de la mollera?*

We tried praying over her and did an egg healing on her for evil eye or *mal de ojo,* and for fright sickness, or *susto,* but nothing has worked. What else can we do? Please help us and keep us in your prayers.

With all due respect to your mother, your baby does not have a *mollera caída*, a fallen fontanel. Your baby is 10 months old and therefore cannot have this condition because her *mollera* has already closed. At birth, there is an area about the size of a quarter on top of the skull above the forehead that has yet to close the soft spot, or fontanel.

After birth, it takes the skull bone four months to completely enclose the soft spot. After this occurs, there is no longer a soft spot and so there can no longer be a *mollera*, or fontanel, to fall.

Mollera caída, fallen fontanel, is a common folk symptom in which the fallen or sunken fontanel is associated with an irritable and/or hungry baby. This condition is usually called *caída de la mollera* but that is technically incorrect. It's actually vice versa, an infant who is sickly, dehydrated and not nursing adequately, will lose body weight and water weight causing the fontanels to sink or fall.

A *mollera caída* is usually seen in a baby suffering from intestinal dysentery or another illness which causes the infant to not breast or bottle feed. The hungry child becomes extremely irritable and refuses to respond to nursing. Folk beliefs hold that the fontanel, or mollera, must be reset, and pulled outward to its normal position. This is a common folk illness and is generally achieved by holding the baby upside down and tapping gently on the bottom of the feet while pressing gently down on the palate with one's thumb. If the pressure "pops" the fontanel back to its normal position, then the baby is once again able to nurse without pain. An infant that refuses to be nursed and has diarrhea, must be taken to a medical doctor immediately.

BABY CRIES IN THE WOMB
LLANTO DEL BEBÉ

Grandmother has a grand daughter who is pregnant and has heard her baby cry from inside the womb. Could there be something wrong with the baby? We are afraid to say anything to the doctor again because when we mentioned it to her, she did not understand us. She did not even believe us and she looked at us as if we were crazy!

In the traditional *Hispanic* culture, it has been my experience and belief than an unborn baby can cry in the mother's womb. While I have never heard it myself, many people have told me that it is true.

In Hispanic culture, we are taught to believe that when a baby cries from within the mother's womb, that it is a sign that the child is going to be born with a gift or *don* from God. I hope and pray that this is of some consolation and comfort.

Every culture has unique, if not magical, beliefs about pregnancy and birth. They include the belief about what influences the fetus and what special qualities the fetus will display as an adult.

Few parents have heard their fetus cry in the womb, but those who have, attribute special spiritual abilities to these unique children. The *Hispanic* culture uses the metaphor "Gift from God" to describe these blessed children and fervently believe that they're destined to be clairvoyants and/or healers with a very special gift.

Grandmother, can a baby be *asustado/a* or frightened, before birth. My niece went through a traumatic event when she was about eight months pregnant. Could this have affected the baby in any way? We know that the baby shudders while she is sleeping. Please let me know what grandmother thinks.

I also have a great-niece that I believe needs to be cured for *susto*. Grandmother used to do it for us and of course no one thought to write down the instructions to cure *susto* before she died.

I know I need lime, called *cal* in Spanish, and mugwort, called *estafiate*, and that it is supposed to be done for three days. Are there special days when it is supposed to be done, and what about prayers?

I am of the opinion that whatever affects the pregnant mother physically and psychologically also affects the unborn child to some degree physically or emotionally. The effects may be even greater where there has been a traumatic event, physical, emotional or psychological.

In some traditional folk beliefs, other concerns and symptoms might be present, such as cravings. It is believed that if the expectant mother does not satisfy her craving for a particular food, that the food will affect the unborn child. The fetus may develop hiccup in the womb and will be born with hiccups or will have an open mouth throughout its life. Sometimes these people drool and are called *babosos*.

I do believe a baby can be *asustado,* or frightened, while in the womb. It is the belief of some that if the expectant mother does not receive a treatment for the *susto,* the child will be slow to learn, to speak or will stutter throughout their life.

Shuttering is not considered a symptom or a result of *susto* and is more of a natural involuntary movement of the eyelids or muscles possibly due to dreaming. Another symptom of a person who is *asustado,* is that they will want to sleep all the time.

Grandmother used to have us jump over a hole in the ground filled with water or fire. We would jump over it three times, making the sign of the cross each time and then drop on all fours to drink the water from the hole.

There are many variations on the cure for *susto,* so your grandmother had one and my mother had another. All are effective.

To cure *susto,* I use fresh rue, rosemary and basil to sweep the frightened person. I recommend you look for a *piedra alumbre* or alum rock, at any *hierbería,* herb shop, and sweep the affected individual for nine straight days.

The frightened person should also drink a cup of spearmint tea in the morning during the same nine days and pray to the Archangel Gabriel.

It should be noted here that the home remedies and advice from a *Curandera,* should never serve as a replacement for suggested treatment by a medical doctor. The two treatments may complement each other, but always follow the advice of a physician. It is clear that the visits to grandma will comfort, but aren't meant as substitutes for medical attention.

It is widely believed that the developing fetus is influenced by both natural and supernatural forces. Therefore, the mother must always protect both herself and the fetus.

Espanto is a severe form of fright caused by a ghost or spirit and pregnant women are always mindful not to be startled by them.

Grandmother says that pregnant women should wear a red ribbon around their waists, on their wrists or hang a key amulet pinned to undergarments. These are all designed to protect the baby from harm. The startle is believed to cause the fetus to be *espantado* or scared in the womb.

Espanto might result in the baby being born with a scared look or even twisted face, or unable to speak all together. The baby is also believed to be protected after birth by an *ojo de venado* seed or the deer's eye in the form of an amulet or talisman pinned to the diaper.

BAD AIR
MAL AIRE

My grandmother and my aunts have always said that if you venture out from a hot environment to a cold one without protection or vice versa, you may get sick with the symptoms of a cold or *mal aire.*

Some people are more sensitive to a sudden or drastic change in temperature than others. That is, going from hot to cold or cold to hot. This sudden change of temperature could be caused by going from a cold air-conditioned room to the heat outside or vice versa during the winter.

It can be a shock and very traumatic to the body by going from one extreme to the other. In *Curanderismo,* this is referred to as *agarro* or *pesco un mal aire,* that is, to receive or "catch a bad air."

One cure for *mal aire* or bad air is to place a burning candle on a coin on a person's back or stomach and then to place a drinking glass over the flame. As the flame burns out from lack of oxygen, the glass will press harder on the flesh, forming an airtight seal.

When the glass is removed, it is pulled off gently and with its removal the *mal aire* or intrusive air is believed to be sucked out of the body.

Hispanic folklore believes that a sudden change in the ambient temperature surrounding one's body triggers illness. For example, moving from an air-conditioned room to the warm or hot outdoors is believed to cause a cold, just as going from hot to cold is believed to do the same.

Hispanic will refer to bad air, or *mal aire*, as an invasive predicament affecting the body and the cause of illness.

One ancient technique still practiced by today's *Curanderas* is called *la ventosa*, or cupping. In order to remove the invasive air from the body of the sick person, a coin or another type of metallic object is placed on the skin at the suspected site believed to be influenced by *mal aire*, bad air.

A small candle is then placed on the coin and lighted; a glass or "cup" is then placed over the flame. As the flame flickers down, the skin is gently elevated, thus expelling unwanted air from the body.

The dichotomy of belief between hot and cold foods is also prevalent in *Curanderismo*. In both food and in air, pre-Columbian cultures, as well as Europeans, believed influx retained a physical equilibrium for overall sound health. The slightest change in this balance is believed to cause sickness.

The *Badianus Codex* explains how an illness was precipitated by an imbalance in one's diet. Today, many of the *Curanderas* remedies are efforts to restore and maintain physical and spiritual balance.

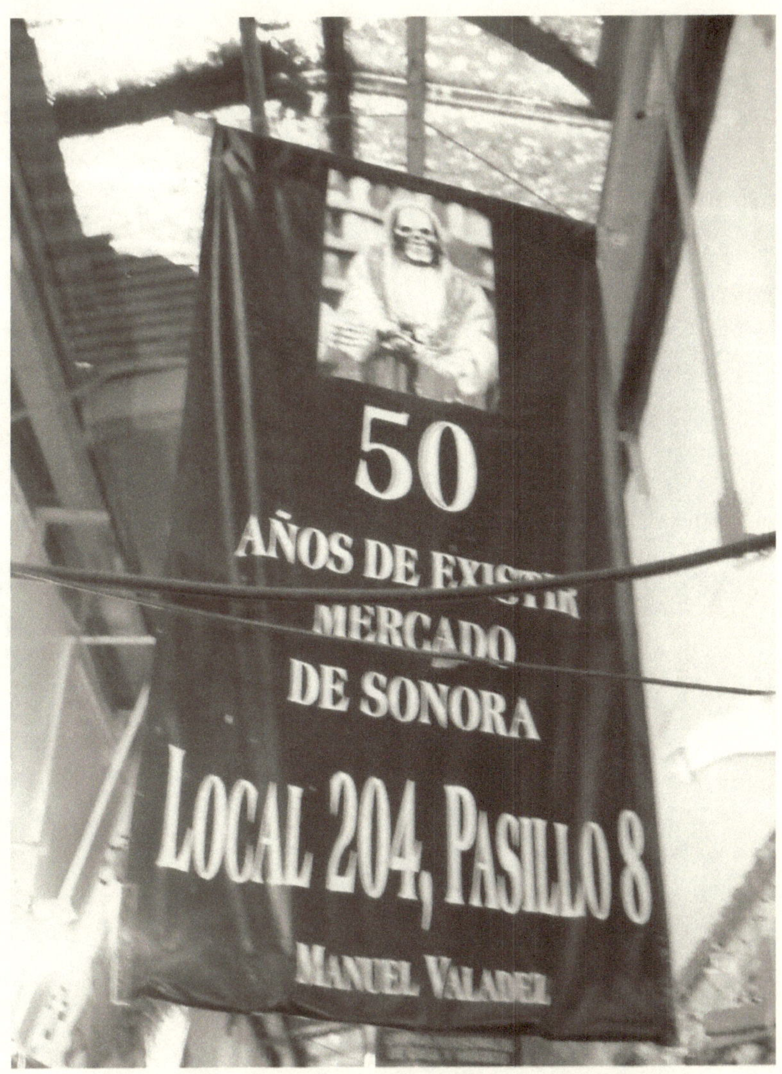

The Mercado Sonora "The Witch's Market in Mexico City Celebrating 50 years of service

Part 2
Remedies of the Frail Mind

THE EVIL EYE
MAL DE OJO

Grandmother, what can be wrong with my child? She was such a happy child but now she is irritable, can't sleep and cries a lot. This started after we attended a party where I know several women were admiring her.

Do you think they might have given her the evil eye? Please pray for her. We have taken her to the doctors and they cannot find anything wrong with her. She is just one year old. She had never gotten sick before. We are scared and don't know what is wrong or what to do. I remember you talking about *mal de ojo or mal ojo* and I even remember being cured for it when I was little.

Let's check her out to see if she has evil eye, *mal de ojo*. Use a fertile chicken egg, one with a live yolk, to do a ritual sweeping, or *limpia*, cleansing on her by rubbing the egg over the child's body, especially her head and her eyes. Be sure to hold the egg in your right hand when you are sweeping her. Begin at her head and proceed down her entire body. Include her arms and legs.

While you are doing the ritual sweeping or *barrida*, you must pray three Apostles' Creeds, or *Credos*.

Another cure comes from an old Mexican belief that women's interior clothing may be used; especially if they are red. When you are giving the *barrida* don't be in a hurry and pray slowly. Place yourself in a spiritual mood and pray to God to remove all evil from her and to heal her.

Crack the eggshell, dropping only the egg yolk but not the shell into a clear glass of water. Examine the egg yolk to see if you can spot what looks like an eye on the yolk or some other identifiable evil shape.

If you can see what looks like an eye, that is a sign that negative energy of the evil eye has been absorbed by the egg from the child. Once this occurs, the afflicted child will settle down from what appears to be a frightening state of illness.

People who practice witchcraft or who want to send the evil eye "back" to the person, who originally sent it will boil the egg and send the evil back to the one who sent it. I don't ever recommend doing this or trying to harm people through a witchcraft spell.

If the child's condition does not improve immediately, the problem is not evil eye and the child should be taken to a physician for further examination.

A red string or a piece of red ribbon with an attached *ojo de venado*, or deer's eye amulet may be tied around the child's wrist or attached to the child's clothing to ward off the evil eye.

The evil eye may unknowingly emanate from seemingly harmless, yet powerful people. Negative energies can come from an unsuspecting person who admires the child, but without even touching the child on the head.

We must always protect an innocent child from the transfer of a strong eye. Touching the child nullifies any energy transmitted by sight. Energies may be transmitted by people and even by animals such as owls, snakes, and cats.

It is clear that a multitude of variations exists in the cure of *mal de ojo* in the practice of *Curanderismo*. One may not prove any better than the other and families maintain their own traditions. In the case of *mal de ojo*, it is important to always protect children from "powerful" glares or stares.

This does not mean that people are evil; some may possess a "strong" or powerful eye that may affect a child by producing fever, restlessness, sleeplessness, and other similar symptoms. If possible, go to the *hierbería* and purchase an *ojo de venado* and pin it on your baby's interior clothing.

ENVY AND JEALOUSY
ENVIDIA Y CELOS

When a person, adult or child, is demonstrating envy or jealousy always treat envy and jealousy by cleansing their person and your home by burning incense such as *myrrh, copal,* and storax or *estoraque,* from the sweet gum tree, also known as liquid amber, mixed with ground coffee beans and a little bit of brown sugar and dry rosemary. Add a few drops of essences of *narciso negro,* tobacco or rose oil, and then grab a handful of the mixture and drop it on the hot coals to cause lots of smoke.

With that, you will begin the ritual of cleansing your home the jealous person and yourself, which will work in removing all the bad and negative forces around you. Be sure to use *narciso negro,* or black narcissus, and mustard drops on the inside of each window and door in your house as protection against envy.

Make an *amulet* against envy by using green cloth. On a Monday, place nine drops of a combination of perfumes against envy, *contra envidia*. Get the recommended perfumes at the *hierbería*. They will sell perfumes to protect you against envy.

Carry the prepared, *preparada*, green cloth amulet on your person for best results. Also, get a specially-prepared white candle from the *hierbería* and every morning before you go to work pass it over your body, saying your special prayer against envy.

Burn a candle on your home altar every evening when you return home. True *Curanderas* establish a meaningful long-term relationship with their clients. Over the years they can become very close and dependent upon each other. They share information about family and friends and look forward to the occasional visit in person.

The *Curandera* does not let the petitioner who is suffering from a mental illness sink deeper into paranoia.

EARACHE FUNNEL
EL CUCURUCHO

Earaches can be very painful and there are a number of things that can cause them. Often air is trapped in the ear, *aire*, or water in the ear. Foreign objects and stopped up ears from colds and influenza can also cause earaches. In older persons, often high blood pressure or sinus problems cause ringing in the ear.

So, as you can see, there can be any number of conditions that cause earaches. It is always recommended that you consult a doctor especially where infections are present and children are involved. Young children are particularly susceptible to chronic ear infections that if left untreated can cause lifelong hearing loss.

One of grandmother's most common home remedies is to place olive oil in the ear or an *unguento*, or unguent, paste made from pig lard covered with a plug of cotton in the ear. Other medicinal plants that are commonly used for earaches include, bay leaf or *laurel;* coriander or *cilantro;* marigold or *calendula;* red sage or *mirto*; and rue or *ruda*.

For generations, grandmothers have been treating earaches with the funnel, or with the *embudo* method. This method is based on the belief that the earache is due to an imbalance of air pressure within the ear caused by trapped air.

Grandmother forms a funnel shape usually from cardboard, placing the narrow end of the funnel slightly into the ear cavity, and then lighting the other end with fire around the edges of the cardboard of the large open end of the funnel.

This remedy is as old as the hills and many of us had this remedy applied to us as children by our grandmothers or aunts. My grandmother performed this cure for me when I was about 8 years old.

However, it is not safe for the funnel procedure to be performed by an inexperienced person and it is never recommended that anyone who is not an expert attempt it.

For example, this procedure must never be done without a container of water handy to extinguish the fire. And it should never be done inside a house.

Once the funneled paper is lit, the fire will burn gradually getting larger and requiring more and more air to burn, thus pulling trapped air out of the inner ear. If there is any excess air causing pressure on the ear, the fire will suck it out causing an audible pop.

Earaches can be traced to a multitude of causes. Both allergies and ear infections cause accumulation of fluids and air trapped in the inner ear; creating a buildup of pressure and pain in the ear. This is very common among children. Many cultures acknowledge that fire sucks out oxygen and air from a higher pressure to a lower pressure.

If air is captured within the inner ear and unable to escape, a paper funnel with the small end placed next to the ear opening with the paper's large end lighted, it draws the trapped air out of the ear; restoring ear-pressure balance, which results in reducing the pain.

SICK BABY
BEBÉ ENFERMITO

Babies sometimes get serious strep infections or maybe the baby has what we call thrush or *algodoncillo* in Spanish. This is a fungus in the mouth that can be easily treated. There are many plant remedies that I use to treat fungus, including, blood root or *sanguinaria*; rue or *ruda*; celandine or *celedonia*; cedar or *cedro*; and tarbush or *ojase*.

Meanwhile, try feeding your baby yogurt sweetened with honey. Give your baby a little bicarbonate of soda to rinse out his mouth and the cotton mouth should clear up quickly. Some of the medicinal plant's grandmothers use for mouth issues include, blackberry or *zarzamora*; sage or *salvia*; flax or *linaza*; oak or *encino;* and orange or *naranja*.

Curanderas always look for both natural and supernatural causes in all childhood illnesses and conditions. Since children are innocent, their illnesses are sometimes thought to be caused by the sin of the parents or other close relatives.

Illnesses occur when the child's fate or luck is altered by something bad the parents did. The child is innocent, but may suffers the consequences. The *Curandera,* is called to reverse bad luck or fortune which will bring about the child's healing. One or both of the parents can become salted, or *salada,* and when this happens their children may be stricken with an illness as a consequence. There are many wonderful resources for child health issues.

RASH
COMEZÓN Y RONCHAS

The itch on my head returns every once in a while, but now it is only very moderate. I do continue using the tomato juice to treat it.

I'm glad that the baths have given you relief for the itch on your body. To continue moving forward with your well-being and to get rid of the itch on your head, you'll have to make a tea with parsley, lavender, *arnica,* lemon grass and common kitchen sage.

Another tea you can take contains cinnamon, or *canela,* with lemon and honey. Prepare a paste made with baked tomatoes and a small amount of liquor, then, rub it all over your body. A boiled liquid made from borage, or *borraja,* can also be applied by rubbing it on the skin to treat sores or *roña.* You could also rub coyote lard, or *manteca de coyote,* mixed with sulfur on the sores.

There are many folk therapies and over-the-counter remedies for irritated, scratchy skin. Rashes and skin issues have many different origins and causes including emotional stress. Always consult a doctor or pharmacist first before you attempt home remedies.

Grandmothers will often prescribe that the body be rubbed with an antibacterial, or antiseptic agent. There are many plants containing these properties including: common radish; and most of the mints or *hierba buena*; all heal or *valeriana*; ambrosia or *hierba amarga*; creosote bush; parsley or *perejil*; dandelion or *diente de leon*; desert bloom or *yerba del pasmo*; horsetail or *cola de caballo*; myrtle or *mirto*; and the two trees, *anacua* and *acacia* or *huizache*. Unguents, or *ungentos*, constituted of barley, or *cebada* achieve the same goal, they produce a soothing, healing salve.

BAREFOOT
LA FRIALDAD

My children love to run around outside barefooted. So, the other day my grandmother warned me that they could get sick doing this, that it was a dangerous practice.

I thought that she was talking about cutting the bottoms of their feet or stepping on a bug, but she said that there were many illnesses that enter the body through the feet, especially when the ground is cold and wet.

Because sometimes my children do get fevers and colds, coughs or other common childhood illnesses for no reason that I can determine. I know they pick up a lot of sicknesses at school as well.

Frialdad, or coldness, is an illness believed to have entered the body through bare feet. This is also believed to be one of the causes of bedwetting in children and even in some adults.

Frialdad is also a concept believed to be one of the reasons that some women are not able to conceive. This type of coldness is referred to as *frialdad de la matriz*, coldness of the uterus, and is an illness believed to have entered the body through bare feet. When this is a diagnosis by the *Curandera* the uterus has to be reheated with teas and massage.

Many *Hispanics* attribute illnesses, misfortunes, suffering and all sorts of problems to having inadvertently stepped on or walked on witchcraft objects which were deliberately placed in their path.

Illnesses or spells are believed to be transferred to the hapless person who touches or comes into contact with contaminated materials that have been used in cleansing healing rituals, recklessly left behind.

My Grandmother is a practitioner of ancient methods of dealing with certain ailments, such as bedwetting. Here is an example, one would take the urine from the bedwetter, and pour it onto hot-clay bricks or red-hot coals.

The urine vaporizes onto the bare feet of the bedwetter who is sitting next to the hot coals. This breaks the coldness, or *frialdad,* in the bladder and brings about the end to bedwetting.

Bedwetting is believed to be a condition that could have come about by the body being exposed to cold temperatures as well. However, drinking excessive fluids near bedtime, or after a trauma, fear, or stressful condition can also cause bedwetting.

Coldness of the uterus is usually treated by massaging the *vientre,* or womb and lower abdomen, with warm olive oil every day. Supernatural illnesses brought about by contact with unclean, demonic, evil spirits and negative energies which have entered the body through the feet will, in all likelihood, require the attention and cleansing of a reputable healer or exorcist if the case warrants it.

In pre-industrial societies it is normal for people to believe that illness enters the body through the feet. This theory is partially true, it has persisted and is passed on generationally. Additionally, it is a common belief that getting wet or walking in water allows illness to enter through the feet.

Many children innocently acquire worms by walking barefooted, especially if there are pets in the yard. Do not rule out having a medical doctor check children for pinworms or hookworms via a stool sample. These are common parasites and enter through bare feet; especially in areas where children coexist with farm animals.

People who live in rural areas around farm animals generally eat pumpkin seeds, or *semilla de calabaza,* a well-known preventive against intestinal parasites or anthelminic, or *antihelmíntico.*

It is well known that when sleeping children grind their teeth, they have worms. This may be verified by checking the child's behind at night when they are asleep and grinding their teeth. Usually, the worms will venture out and can be easily seen.

RHEUMATISM
LAS REUMAS

Grandmother started rubbing her leg and said she was starting to feel a pain in her knee. We told her not to worry that the pain was going to go away but of course it didn't. At times, she says it feels as if though her whole body and all of her joints hurt and she cannot control her legs. She feels that her legs want to move by themselves. At night, she cries because not only the right leg was hurting, but her left knee was starting to hurt as well.

She has been using an ointment, but it takes a while to work, and when it does work it's only for a short while. It really hurts us to see grandmother suffer this way. If its arthritis, I don't know why the over the-counter creams and the medication the doctor gave her do not seem to work.

Grandmother is suffering from *reumas*, that is, arthritis, or rheumatism and there are many folk remedies for these ailments, but this is a normal part of aging and will never completely go away.

I would recommend that you prepare a tea made from garlic cloves simmered in milk. Have her drink the cup of milk for nine consecutive days, especially when she is suffering.

Rub lemon juice on her leg and knee, then rub egg white on her leg when she is in pain.

Grandmother may also make a tea out of lemon grass, *zacate de limón*, and of *salvia* or sage. Have her drink a glass of tomato juice with her meal and then apply tomato juice on a towel and place the towel over the knee and painful area while praying over her. Have her do this twice a day.

Have your grandmother drink cherry juice. Give her an ounce of cherry juice in a glass of water once a day for three straight weeks. Get an extract of *nopal* or cactus leaves, and *linaza* or flax seed from your neighborhood pharmacy, or *hierbería*. If you can't find these ingredients, ask for *linaza* fiber. Use one or the other putting one teaspoon of the fiber in a glass of water. Mix well and give it to her to drink once a day for two straight weeks.

Just to be safe, give your grandmother's home a good *limpia* or spiritual cleansing. Pass a fertile hen's egg over her body. The hen's eggs must be prepared for three days by placing them in a triangular form and by sprinkling or spraying them with perfumes for health and strength. Cleanse her body with the prepared egg every Friday for seven Fridays in a row and her health will return. In order to regain health, perform the ritual that was used to scare away bad energies or witchcraft.

Cleanse her home by performing a *sahumerio* or smoking cleansing ritual, and by asking that all evil and negative forces be cast out of the home.

Her condition is natural, not supernatural or evil. Prepare a tea made by boiling *hierbanís*, anise, and *tumba vaquero*, or morning glory and have her drink one cup of tea a day for seven straight days.

There are a number of different illnesses and conditions that deal with the brain and nerves and each requires a different *remedio*. Some of the most common plants are black mustard or *mostaza negra*; mistletoe or *injerto*; night blooming jasmine or *huele de noche*.

Grandmother must allay the fears of each and every person who wish to affix a supernatural origin to problematic life situations.

While some persons may want to blame witchcraft or evil origins to every situation they encounter, it is unrealistic to believe witchcraft is responsible for every negative health condition in our lives.

Grandmothers will often use a number of personally, acquired and learned healing techniques. These include both actual and spiritual surgery, as well as blowing into the body, sucking out of the patient's body and spiritually transferring illness or objects from a patient to the healer.

As a result, Grandmothers can often be taken ill through these processes and will go through a period of rest and the cleansing of their bodies before they may return to full health. During the time she is suffering she cannot heal.

PREGNANCY AND BIRTH
ENCINTA Y DAR A LUZ

One of the most important issues in every family is the ability to get pregnant and maintain a pregnancy to term followed by a normal delivery. Sometimes this is very difficult and couples endure years or a lifetime without being able to conceive. This causes great stress in the family, especially with the couple's parents who want a grandchild.

It is believed that the female reproductive organs are cold and must be heated in order for conception to take place. In Hispanic culture, people learn that illness and many health conditions are caused by imbalances in the body; the by-products of improper foods with hot versus cold properties.

A tea of *damiana* or *turnera diffusa,* and others which should be taken in the morning and at night. This usually warms the reproductive system which when heated promotes pregnancy and the woman gets pregnant in most cases. Special massages with olive oil or other specially prepared oils are usually required of the lower abdomen area as well. This is to make sure that all of the organs are in their proper location and condition as well as to heat them.

One of the by-products of pregnancy is the production of gas in the intestines and this may be controlled with a tea made from sage or yarrow. This *carminativo,* or carminative, will also reduce the abdominal discomfort.

Many grandmothers will also treat pregnant women with olive oil which acts as a cathartic, or *catártico,* purgative or *purga* used to clean out the female digestive system.

The family usually wants to determine the gender of the baby and there are many techniques for determining the sex of the unborn baby. The women of the family will hold a red string with a needle dangling over the belly of the expectant mother. If the needle rotates clockwise, that indicates the baby will be a boy and if it rotates counter-clockwise it indicates a girl.

Protecting the unborn and developing baby from outside negative forces is also very important. For example, the unborn baby should never be exposed to unusual lunar phenomenon such as a lunar eclipse because this is believed to cause a deformity in the fetus. To prevent this, *talismans* and amulets are worn under clothing to protect the developing baby.

These are just a few of the hundreds of remedies and beliefs that exist and that we utilize during the various stages leading up to pregnancy, during pregnancy, during and after delivery.

And never forget that when a mother is pregnant, it will affect the behavior and moods of existing small children who will become jealous of the new baby, especially when children are removed from their mother's breast to make room for the newly arrived baby.

Additionally, when a baby is sad, he or she is said to be *chipil,* which means that they are jealous of the new baby who displaced them. Conditions surrounding pregnancy and birth are among the most common and important in human populations.

Grandmothers know that they must be prepared to treat these conditions with all of their time-tested remedies.

Herbal teas, massages, magical protections and prayers to the appropriate saint are all necessary to ensure a positive outcome of pregnancy and birth. These cautions are just as important to all female family members as they are to the expectant mother.

There are many herbal teas that assist pregnancy. Many also are used to assist the reproductive system in flushing lingering menstrual fluids. This is called an emmenagogue, or *emenagogo.* Yarrow or *milenrama* is commonly used for this. Pregnancy also causes water weight gain or edema.

An entire category of medicinal plants exists, such as borage, or *borraja*, used to promote the generous flow of breast milk after birth. These herbs are called galactogogues, or *galactagogos*, because they promote and enhance the production of breast milk.

Ailments and illnesses come and go. It's trendy to attribute a cure to a medicinal plant or a prescribed medicine. However, one must be cautious! In addition to all of the popular folk medicines, the *Curandera* should always refer a person to a physician or clinic which specializes in nurse-midwife assisted births. Regarding pregnancy and birth the person should ask for advice from both the doctor and the *Curandera*.

DISOBEDIENT CHILD
EL HIJO PRÓDIGO

Grandmother, my son is a recovering drug addict and alcoholic. He rarely works, but has recently quit all his addictions. But because he doesn't work, he is always asleep or in a bad mood. I think that he is in a deep depression.

Grandmother what can I do to help him, what do you recommend? I know he is in God's hands but I also believe that it is my responsibility to seek spiritual help and corporal healing for him, and that our Lord Almighty will help him not to give up on life. I know that God has charged me to continue to support my son, but I need your help.

Esteemed granddaughter, there is no doubt that you are a saint. God will continue to give you strength, health, and valor so that the cross you carry won't be so heavy.

Please boil creosote bush or *gobernadora*, and bathe your son with the water for seven straight days. Be sure to immerse his entire body including his head in the water.

You can also treat your son's depression with *plantas medicinales* such desert anemone or *hierba mansa*; persimmon or *nispero*; linden or *Tila*, and rue or *ruda*.

I also ask you to pray the prayer of the *Lost Boy*, *Niño Perdido* which is from a little boy who appeared in the Mexican state of *Guanajuato* many years ago. He is different from the boy Jesus who stayed in the temple.

There are no books about the Lost Boy or *Niño Perdido*, only an *estampa* or holy card. Give yourself a healing spiritual bath with the water of *romero*, or rosemary, for seven consecutive Fridays. God will give you valor and patience.

Then, give your son a spiritual cleansing with a crucifix and a handful of fresh herbs of *albahaca*, basil, *pirul*, California pepper, *romero*, rosemary, and *ruda*, rue. Also, give yourselves cleansings with herbs for seven straight Mondays or Fridays. Do this, while you pray asking God to fulfill your prayers.

Evil will always try to overwhelm good. I am very happy to know that your son has abandoned the repulsive vices of drugs and alcohol. You must continue with his spiritual healing. It is also possible that he is traumatized by some past shock or some other ailment. You may have to treat him for *susto*. We need to struggle on through life because where there is bad, there is also good. Someone once said, "For a mother there is no bad son."

Scant factual information exists about the *Niño Perdido*, the lost child. There is a popular tale about a child who lost his mother. At some time in the early 20th century, the followers of the *Niño Perdido* moved the image into the *barrios* south of San Antonio, Texas. It has survived there to this day.

The *Niño Perdido* has become the *Tejano* patron saint for mothers; mostly for those with sons and daughters who are away at war. Prayers are offered to the *Niño Perdido* to return a son or daughter safely home from overseas.

The *Curandera* reaches deep into the core of her faith. The *Hispanic* population deeply reveres Saint Jude, or *San Judás Tadeo,* and his ability to resolve their most impossible cases.

The *Curandera* senses the desperation in this person's voice, and that time is quickly elapsing for this family. Failure to resolve their issues will evolve into the next generation and literally destroy its spirit.

Prayer is the answer which must be combined with a practical strategy to primarily resuscitate family communication, followed by unity and participation.

HUMORAL THEORY
TEORÍA HUMORAL

Grandmother says that I should be concerned about the hot and cold nature of the foods I eat. What exactly is a hot food or a cold food? At first, I thought grandmother was talking about the temperature of the foods, but then I quickly learned they were talking about the properties the food is believed to have.

Foods, including most meats, grease or lard, eggs and corn are considered to have hot properties, they promote growth and they accelerate body functions. Sometimes this is good and they are needed, but other times not.

Cold foods include most fresh vegetables and fruits, either eaten fresh or in the form of a soup, dairy products, fish and chicken. The temperature of the soup does not influence that the food is a cold or hot food.

Outside conditions are also very important. If a child is affected by rapid changes in temperature by going from hot too cold without protection, they will develop a runny nose and possibly a cold. We call this condition *pasmo*, and we know it is not a virus and can be resolved by administering hot foods like chicken soup, or *sopa*, and protection from cold floors and walls. If the child has a fever along with the runny nose, then a tea of *borraja*, or borage, or *muicle*, also called Mexican honeysuckle, or a variety of other fever-reducing plants will work to reduce the fever. Remember, that a feverish person must be brought back into balance before they can recover.

PRAYING FOR GOOD HEALTH
ORANDO

Grandmother I have been saying the prayers you gave me for weeks. "Oh, powerful spirit of the Patron Saint." "Oh, Divine Spirit" pray for us. However, I am not sure that I am saying it correctly or at the right time or using the correct candles for these prayers. I am also not sure what the proper situations are for each candle and each prayer.

I want to pray that I regain my confidence and that my strength returns to me. I pray that I will be sure to make the right decisions. I want to pray for my husband so that he can stop getting so angry and upset at work. I want to pray that the people who he works with will stop bothering him and will leave him alone. I want to pray for my sister's behavior to improve. I want to pray that she will respect her elders and do as she is told and that she will find a renewed interest in school, work and family. I get so upset with her because she is so disrespectful. Grandmother, please continue to pray for me to have patience with her and to help my family.

There is a special time for prayer, and the best time is when there is a special need. Prayer must come from within you, from the heart. There is prayer for the self that should be recited alone. This is a private, personal prayer. There is also open, public prayer, and there are prayers for others. There are thankful prayers of gratitude. Also, prayer is most sacred and most powerful when one is fasting.

The Lord teaches that when two or more come together in His Holy name, He is there amongst you. *Curanderas* who work in the spiritual realm believe that the special time for prayer is at 3 a.m.

Some form of prayer has always been an integral part of healing rituals. In colonial Mexico professionals are hired called ensalmadores were who are believed to heal by reciting the Psalms. Today, *Curanderas* frequently ask their clients to pray certain Psalms.

Prayers are accepted anytime they are offered. *Curanderas* recommend specific prayers and candles for certain situations, but most people feel greatly relieved and improved by any prayer whenever it is recited for them.

Grandmother mentions that it is common to pray at 3 a.m., but this is principally a practice of the spiritist who believes that the veil between the physical world and the spirit world is thinnest at that hour.

GRANT ME STRENGTH
FORTALÉCEME

I wish with all my heart that God will give you spiritual strength, so that you may continue to guide us and help us. I am praying for you. Bathe with the water of *ruda*, rue, *albahaca*, basil, *romero* rosemary. I feel desperate, and the fear of losing my job fills me with many doubts and emotional instability. I want to ask the Saints for strength, light and support to continue with the cycle of life, as God mandates. I have a profession and it has gone badly for me lately. I am convinced that I am bewitched, but I have faith and believe in miracles.

You should burn *copal* incense in your home for seven straight Fridays while praying the Our Father. Also, if you can, bathe with herbs. Always bathe on a Friday. Boil *ruda*, rue, *romero*, rosemary and *albahaca*, basil, and bathe with the water. The night before, strain your tea and then reheat it and bathe for seven consecutive Fridays praying the Hail Mary seven times. Say the prayer to the Holy Trinity to obtain and maintain a good job.

I am pleased that you have started your herbal-healing baths. I recognize that you have supernatural obstacles that stand in your way, but be strong because they will not win out over you. You must have faith and be more stubborn than those who would see you fail.

Also, it is critical that you religiously complete your bathing rituals on Fridays as I asked. No other day will complete the requirements for the ritual and will negate its effects. You must understand that this is a matter of ritual and requires consistency. If you can maintain discipline, the Holy Spirit will provide you with all you need to live happy and content.

When you take these baths on the seven straight Fridays, be sure to also invoke the sacred name of Saint Michael the Archangel and ask for his protection. Invoke Saint Rafael the Archangel and ask him for health of body, soul and spirit. Invoke Saint Gabriel the Archangel and ask him for happiness. After your baths with herb water, say the prayers to the saints.

Your situation is like a salacious assault, or wrongdoing, or like a curse that has befallen you and your life. But finally, if you do as grandmother asks, you will win out over evil.

Within the pantheon of helpful spirits and entities, the archangels are considered the most powerful and are called upon for all sorts of difficult cases. There are many other entities also believed to intercede for us in our times of need.

For example, the Archangel Rafael is the archangel of healing, pray to him for a special intercession.

Spiritual baths and other prescribed regimens may be followed closely but don't necessarily have to be adhered to exactly unless they are parts of magical spells. In those cases, they must be followed exactly or they will not work. In this book grandmother has offered examples of many different saints to pray to and rituals that can be performed for a new intercession.

SPIRITUAL ASSISTANCE
AYUDA ESPIRITUAL

I'm new at this, but I am confident now more than ever that you can help me. I have been looking for spiritual help for a long time since things aren't going good for me.

My life is in a cycle that I can't seem to get out of. First, my life seems to get better for a little bit, but then, just as fast, it turns around to the negative again. I have looked for help but haven't found it. I know what is happening to me, but I can't find the solution. Grandmother I hope you can help me.

You have always been and continue to be, high and mighty, and at the same time not very trustful. Perhaps you have a reason. You have always looked for help and have come out being betrayed. Now everything looks too real and true to you. You don't know whether to believe in God or not. You find yourself very confused. I don't blame you. The cure you seek is in your own hands. In order for you to get rid of all your doubts it is totally up to you.

Your real problem is that you have no faith in God. Start to meditate on the Lord. Do this at three in the morning every day in prayer.

Also, do it every night for an hour until the spirit of God reveals Himself to you. Fast in the mornings for 40 straight days.

Also, read Psalm 23 at noon for 40 consecutive days. After doing this, everything will clear up for you. Your true path will be revealed to you.

People who have healing power are often referred to *Curanderas* by their family and friends, without ever having consulted one before. The physical appearance of the *Curandera* or grandmother's, consulting room, or *consultorio,* as well as their rituals may seem extremely bizarre to a first timer.

First impressions and the building of confidence are difficult. It takes time but definitely produces positive results. Frequently, people seek simple solutions to complex personal problems, relying on others instead of making meaningful changes in their lives. "God helps he who helps himself."

The *Curandera* can offer spiritual support but not for the person looking for a quick fix. The individual must take the situation seriously. There is no magical pill to transform life into a dream. Persons who refuse to confront the enemy within themselves and are so self-centered that to them help means sucking all the energy out of the healer who offers it, will ultimately fail.

Ask a Curandera to perform a year end ritual for you. First ask for a reading with La Baraja, or Tarot cards. For hundreds of years, it has been the custom to eat twelve grapes at midnight to clear away bad forces from you. Get a hand full of lentils from the grocery store and place them around your house and carry some in your pocket or purse. This ritual will assist you in clearing away bad energies which may be lingering around you.

Always give your home a *limpia* or *sahumerio* at the beginning of each year. Pray the Apostle's Creed as you perform the cleansing.

OLD-FASHIONED
ABUELITA ANTICUADA

Ever since I was a little girl, I remember my grandmother telling me about foods that we can eat and cannot eat at different times in life and I really never understood why. She said that where she was from in Mexico, everyone takes into consideration the hot and cold nature of foods.

My grandmother raised me because my mother was not around and I don't want to offend her so I listened, I don't want to just obey; I want to understand. When I was in school, I asked my teachers about my grandmother's beliefs, but they didn't know and just shrugged their shoulders.

Now I am going to have a baby and I asked my doctor about what my grandmother is telling me and they just say these are crazy old wife's tales from Mexico. These doctors didn't understand either.

I still live with my grandmother and she simply won't let me eat certain foods because she says they will harm the baby. I want to respect my grandmother, but I also want to understand her beliefs.

You have every right to understand. Both my maternal and my paternal grandmothers had large families, and I am the eldest of 10 in our family. All my aunts and uncles also have large families. Being raised around large families, I know very well of your grandmother's advice regarding food. I have heard it my whole life and people frequently ask about it.

She is telling you about how to be careful with what are called the hot and cold qualities of foods not the temperature of food.

In *Hispanic* culture and in others, there are many beliefs about what foods should be eaten or avoided during pregnancy. From grandma's and my *Curandera's* view, foods prepared in vinegar or with any kind of chili, hot sauces or spices are thought to have hot qualities and are not appropriate for pregnant women.

Also, some meats like pork should be avoided because it is a hot food while chicken is a cold food. These foods, which raise the body's temperature, are not believed to be good for the developing baby or the mother.

Likewise, when the body is hot from illness or fever, it is thought that you can bring down the temperature by giving bland or cold foods. A vegetable soup, for example, is cold. There is no harm in any of this and if it makes your grandmother happy, then why not "humor" her?

Always consult your physician and ask them to tell you about hot-and-cold food taboos and humoral theory. Be sure to go to your prenatal checkups, but you are correct to ask questions and expect helpful answers.

Grandmother is not necessarily old fashioned, but she is operating in another cultural mode that should be comprehended, and most importantly respected.

There are many world cultures today that continue the practice of food taboos associated with pregnancy and birth, as well as with different disease states. These taboos frequently find their ways into the United States health-care delivery system.

In *Hispanic* culture, it is widely known that women are told to eat bananas and avocados during their menstrual cycles in order to ease distress.

It's medically documented that diet influences endometriosis which may be linked to different types of behavioral changes. Many cultures know this from untold generations of word-of-mouth experiences passed down from mothers to daughters.

High blood pressure is usually treated with several capsules of garlic, always follow the instructions. This is if you do not suffer from gastric ulcers or indigestion. I treat headaches with numerous plants and combinations of plants.

For example, the ash tree or *sauz*; but also, aspen or *alamo*; feverfew or *altamisa;* honeysuckle or *muicle;* marigold or *calendula*; hibiscus or flor *de Jamaica*; kidneywort or *hepática;* mint bee balm or oregano; and purple sage or *cenizo*, and many others can be used.

Most commonly, I ask people to take *toronjil*, Mexican giant hyssop, tea, one cup a day. For your migraines and all headaches, you may regularly drink a tea made of hackberry bark, *palo blanco*, or from willow or *sauz*.

Find the tea of this sacred bark to clean your digestive system with the corn silk and the *hierba de la hormiga*, ant herb, or pink windmills, to wash out urinary ducts.

After detoxifying your body, nourish yourself with the most correct diet and take vitamins and minerals for strength. What is positive is that you are aware of your ills and don't put off doing what grandmother recommends.

HERBAL MEDICINE
PLANTAS MEDICINALES

There are hundreds of medicinal plants proven to effectively treat numerous illnesses. For example, basil or *albahaca* has various qualities, uses, virtues, faculties and powers. It has also been used as a spice for cooking, as an herb for making tea to calm the nerves, tea to help you sleep, used also as an aromatic fragrance, used in cleansing the spirit, to cure the soul from fright or *susto*, past fright *susto pasado*, or trauma.

It's also used in spiritual baths to rid negative energies, for good luck against bad currents and to draw money, as an extract, as perfume, as oil used to massage injuries, and also used as incense for self-cleansing and cleansing businesses, and your home. In many ways, it is one of the "master" herbs.

If you have a urinary tract infection, take a tea made from ant herb, or *hierba de la hormiga*, and corn silk.

CANDLES
LAS VELAS SIRVEN

It is always a good practice to keep candles in the home and not to replace candles until they no longer smoke. While the candle smokes, it is doing its job of cleansing and healing. It's okay that the candle burns fast and has a high flame, and that it is smoking.

Be very careful to not let the glass crack and cause a fire. Keep it in a dish with a little water just in case it breaks or burns all the way down, so that it won't cause a fire in your home. Also, if there is a price tag on the bottom of the glass, remove it. This is one of the fire hazards when the candle burns down.

Scare bad vibes and energies away from you with candle magic. Get two yellow candles and one red from the hierbería as well as seven goat perfume, *siete machos*. First sprinkle the siete machos on the three candles. Then give yourself a full body limpia from head to toe using the candles. Remember to hold them in your right hand. Place the candles in a glass and add rum. Light incense to clear out any negative energies. Place the three candles in the form of a triangle Call upon the Archangels to assist you and pray the Holy Mary and the Our Father once a day until the candles burn out. Throw the remains of the candles out of your house and bathe in the water and rum that remains. Expect to have cleared out all negative energy from your life and home.

Always interpret your burned candles or have someone who is competent and whom you have confidence in to do it for you. First of all there are always candles that wont light and that is because their spiritual space is blocked. If your candle weeps wax that means that there is something out of order, place the candle in another location. If the candle blows out easily this is a good sign that your issues have been resolved. You are very fortunate if your candle burns down without leaving any trace of wax. This indicates that your petition has been accepted.

If your candle has a high and vigorous flame then it is working in your favor. Conversely a small flame that struggles to stay lit is having a hard time working in your favor. Be sure to place your candle around religious objects.

Of course, a blue flame is the most positive worker. A yellow flame is a sign that the job is more difficult. A large white flame indicates that the angels and Saints are assisting you to achieve your desired outcome. Flames may also sizzle in which case the candle is having problems resolving your issue. Pray in order to give the flame strength.

STRONG DREAM MAN
EL SOÑADOR

Very often people seeking political office will visits grandmother and other *Curanderas*. When I first announced my candidacy, I told everyone that I would run on my merits, and not say anything bad about my opponent, leaving the decision to the voters.

But now, I have been warned that my opponent, who is part of the local political machine, has hired a witch or *bruja,* to not only defeat me, but to harm me and my political family.

Quite frankly I'm worried about this because I want to do the right thing and I don't want any problems. My opponent fears my popularity and my honesty. I have been told that there is a *"strong dream man,"* a noted *curandero,* living near me who can help me to reverse any witchcraft spell that has been done to me.

Last night, a white dove appeared in my dream and landed on my hands and I felt that was a good sign. My kids found something ugly in our yard and, today one of my campaign workers suggested that I contact my you, grandmother.

I highly recommend that you consult a *Curandera* because I know the strong dream man works with the spirits of light and not of darkness. Your dream of a white dove landing on your open hands is a revelation of the gift of the Holy Spirit.

The Holy Spirit is anointing your hands with the Divine healing power of God. You can expect that you will receive many more spiritual dream messages, and that over time they will reveal a spiritual path for you to take in your life.

You will win your campaign, but you will have to always be protected spiritually from here on out. Evil never forgets. Thank you, grandmother, I won my election.

During your campaign keep a journal by your bed and write down each dream you have. Before long, a pattern will emerge telling you what your opponent is trying to do to you.

I sense that you are indeed being worked by a witch and that you need spiritual assistance from the strong dream man. The strong dream man is a renowned shaman who will go into a trance and with his spirit out of his body he will fly to where they are working you and literally see what is being done to you. Then he will tell what you have to do to reverse it.

BAD LUCK
LA MALA SUERTE

Grandmother, we would be ever so grateful if you could give us some advice on what to do with the sudden black cloud that we have hanging over us. My husband broke his left wrist, and went back to work on light duty, then a few weeks later he broke his right ankle and has been out of work since then.

We need help financially. We have bills to pay and we need better health. I have heard rumors from people who work at the plant where he works, and they say that the company is not planning to give him his job back. I don't see how that can happen, but I guess it can.

The woman that he works with is very evil and I think she is causing all this because he would not sleep with her. No one knows what she is capable of doing to us.

I am severely depressed. I don't even feel like getting out of bed every day. The joy has gone out of my life. I am living one day at a time. Is there any hope for us? Something is seriously wrong with me; I have no energy whatsoever. One of my friends told me this is a symptom of depression.

There are still negative energies around you, which have caused someone to be jealous of you or to envy you, *envidia*.

Grandmother recommends that you boil rosemary, basil and rue, and to strain the herbs from the boiled water and then to add one-half cup of honey to the water and for both you and your husband to bathe in the water.

NERVOUS BREAKDOWN
ATAQUE DE NERVIOS

Grandmother, I think I have been given the evil eye, mal *de ojo*? My girlfriend says that I am having a nervous breakdown, or what is called *ataque de nervios*.

Begin a spiritual cleansing of your home by burning incense such as *copal* and sprinkling *Siete Machos* and bathe with orange blossom water and Holy Water.

The most traditional herb for calming the nerves is linden tea, or *té de Tila*. There are many others including: wormseed or *epazote*; poppy or *amapola;* sweet basil or *albahaca*; coriander or *cilantro*; giant hyssop or *toronjil;* lemon balm or *abejera;* persimmon or *nispero*; violet or violeta; and white sapote or *zapote blanco.*

Grandmother says that this young man is *asustado*, he has some level of fright sickness. At some point in the past, he must have suffered a scare or a startle which may have chased some segment of his spirit out of his body. His body is longing for its return.

The missing part of the spirit can only be reunited with the body if the appropriate prayers and rituals are performed coaxing the spirit back into the boy's body to make him whole again.

Susto, or fright sickness, can also be a form of post-traumatic stress disorder (PTSD) which is directly traced to an experience or events that impacted the person years ago.

Susto can also occur during a pregnancy. The fetus is believed to experience the same emotions and trauma as the mother during pregnancy. Nervous breakdown or *ataque de nervios* is a very common occurrence and folk diagnosis or culture-bound syndrome in *Hispanic* populations. In reality, it's often a diagnosis of many conditions lumped into a singular concept referred to as "*nervios*."

The most popular tranquilizer, or *tranquilazador,* for anxiety, or *ansiedad,* is *té de tila,* or linden tea, and *marrubio,* or horehound. Sedatives, or *sedantes,* and soporifics or *soporíficos,* and herbs for sleeplessness or insomnia, insomnia, such as the giant hyssop, or *toronjil,* and *albahaca* are used to treat sleeplessness.

The following are culture-bound syndromes identified in the DSM-IV and discussed extensively in this book: *ataque de nervios*; *bilis* and *cólera (not to be confused with cholera) or muínas; locura; mal de ojo; nervios; spell or trabajo; and susto.*

BAD DREAM
PESADILLA

Grandmother it's been three years since my divorce and since then, my life has become a nightmare, causing me deep emotional problems. I have lost everything: my health, my money, my house, and my job. I just can't seem to get ahead. I wish you could tell me if it's an evil spirit which has latched onto me or if it's simply life.

Do you know what a scapular, or *escapulario,* is? I am sure that you have seen people who wear small colored wool pieces of cloth around their necks. They can be brown, or black, or red, or green and other colors depending on their intended purpose, saint or organization. It is a well-known fact that scapulars are miraculous and when the proper one is worn, the patron saint of the scapular will sometimes grant you an ordinarily unattainable goal.

I recommend that you go to any religious store and purchase a green scapular dedicated to the Immaculate Heart of Mary. Pray to our Mother Mary to resolve your family problems and to restore your health and happiness.

Severe psychological and emotional problems often produce equally impactful physical symptoms. The concept of witchcraft is such an integral concept in *Hispanic* life and culture that it is almost always considered a cause before emotional problems surface. When people are facing difficult situations, emotional symptoms may be ruled out as reasons for illness.

Many of life's daily challenges are actually teaching tools which make us stronger and stimulate us to use our faith and common sense. Without life's ups and downs, many persons would become complacent and suffer a gradual loss of compassion.

In this most difficult and desperate case, grandmother recommends that her family wear a green scapular. Scapulars were worn by monks and other religious figures during the middle-ages. They were popularized by lay or third orders to reflect devotion and affiliation to a confraternity, or *cofradía*.

Scapulars are worn when individuals require special miracles and/or dedicate a novena to a saint for their personal intentions and needs.

NIGHTMARES
PESADIAS

Grandmother said that she noticed that the baby was having nightmares and thought that the baby was scared in his sleep, or had *sueño asustado*. This behavior is very unlike him since he is a very good-natured baby and sleeps well. How do I cure him?

Grandmother is correct and it is good that you are listening to her. A part of his spirit was scared out of him for some reason and must be coaxed back to make him whole again.

Children who are very bright and alert begin to watch their parents at a very early age. If they see conflict between them, they become scared. I believe that is what has happened to your baby boy.

Don't fight or yell in front of your child. In the long run, you can hurt him and warp his behavior. Their fears become part of their permanent personalities, their souls, spirits and their subconscious minds.

Grandmother says, go to the *hierbería* and buy a large white candle called a *cirio*. Buy one that is not in a glass container. Also, buy three small alum rocks, or *piedras alumbre*. The store will probably have fresh basil, or *albahaca*, or can tell you where to buy it. You will also need green rubbing alcohol, aspirin and tobacco.

For three days in a row and, at precisely the same time every day, give your baby a ritual cleansing, first with the basil and then with the *piedra alumbre*.

Be sure to cleanse the baby from head to toe while doing this. Sweep downward holding all items used to cleanse in your right hand.

Light the white candle. The candle will let you know if the cure is working. If it burns without smoking, then the cure is working. As long as it smokes, more cleansing is required.

Mix a small amount of the alcohol with one or two aspirins and use this mixture to make the cross on his hands, arms, legs and feet at the bending points; wrist, elbow and the back of the neck. While you make the sign of the cross on him, gently puff tobacco smoke from a cigar around his head but not in his face.

Be sure to recite three Our Fathers, *Padre Nuestro,* or three Apostles' Creeds, *Credos.* After the first day, you should begin to see an improvement in his behavior and he should sleep better as well. By the second day, if he really is *asustado,* the lighted candle should begin to crackle while you are cleansing him, letting you know that something is happening.

By the third treatment, he should be a happy baby boy once again and totally cured. At the end of the three days, take the used alum rocks outside and carefully burn them in a small can.

Young children are most susceptible to a scare by their new or unknown experiences early in their lives. For example, newborns are sensitive to noise and motion, light and dark as well as hot and cold.

All these aforementioned factors are equivalent to parents in their oblivious mode of incessant arguing and shouting, making their baby feel unsafe in the world.

However, fright, or *susto*, is also known to occur during pregnancy and affect the developing fetus.

The earliest medical texts available to us from the old and new worlds suggest many unpredictable situations during pregnancy which adversely affect the developing fetus. It is also commonly believed that factors which impact the pregnant mother or may scare her, could affect the fetus in a negative way.

If the fetus is believed to be scared while in the mother's womb, it is capable of violent shakes and can even cry in the womb.

These are all ominous signs in the *Hispanic* world and indicate that something adverse is happening or could happen to the developing baby. The result could be something as benign as a birthmark or as serious as a birth defect.

ECLIPSE OF THE MOON
ECLIPSE DE LUNA

My baby was delivered by a midwife, or *partera*. I went to this special birthing center because they specialize in *Hispanic* cultural beliefs. They explained to me that they were going to teach me the "old ways" and I would just love it.

For the first time in my life, I felt connected to something, even though I didn't always understand what they were telling me. And, in fact, they don't really know or understand the origins for a lot of the things they taught me.

Help me to understand the influence of the moon on development and why we believe that moonbeams and eclipses of the moon can hurt the baby before it is born?

The moon is associated with both the natural and the supernatural influences and phenomena of prenatal development. Some believe that the moon is a heavenly body with magical or spiritual qualities. Others hold it to be virtuous and full of mystical powers.

Hispanics believe that if an expectant mother does not protect the developing fetus from moonlight, when the moon is full there could be serious consequences to the child's well-being and the child runs the risk of being born deformed. People say that the moon will eat, or *comer,* the baby while in the womb if the moonbeams fall on the pregnant mother.

This is especially true during a lunar eclipse when pregnant women should protect themselves by not going outside or standing in front windows where the moon is fully visible.

To protect the baby and prevent the moon from eating away at an unborn baby, the expectant mother should attach a safety pin or a key to her clothes directly over her stomach. The mother-to-be should also wear red undergarments or tie a red ribbon around her body over her stomach to protect the unborn baby.

The belief that the stars and moon affect outcomes of conception and determine behavioral characteristics of the unborn can be traced back to the beginning of time.

There are many ancient beliefs from all cultures about the harmful nature of moonbeams on the developing fetus. The belief that moonbeams "falling" upon the unprotected belly of a pregnant woman will deform a fetus is found in many ancient texts. Protect your unborn baby.

NIGHT DEW
EL SERENO MALO

I am a young Hispanic and I have a newborn baby. I am trying to be a good mother, but I don't know how to do it. Everyone I speak to seems to have a better idea about how I should raise my baby, and what is good and what is bad.

I don't know who to believe and I hope you can help me. On the issue of covering up the baby's head outdoors, I am told that the baby's head needs to be kept warm because it loses heat right away.

Also, I am told never to let the evening dew or *sereno* fall on the baby's head because that will make him sick. Can you please help me to understand and what to believe or not to believe?

The condition known as *serenar* refers to illnesses influenced by evening dew, or *sereno.* This is a concern with many *Hispanics* who have babies. The belief is that the baby should never be exposed to evening dew. If the baby must be taken out at night, the baby's head should always be covered because it is the most vulnerable place on the body. If the child is exposed to the *sereno,* the child may become susceptible to illness.

The baby who becomes *serenado* may suffer chills, body pains and headaches, and the child's stool will be greenish in color. Additionally, it is believed that the child or baby may become ill if dressed with clothes left out overnight in the evening dew.

Chamomile tea is often boiled in milk and given to children as a remedy for this condition.

All cultures swaddle newborn infants and know to keep them covered up. This is especially true of their heads. Grandmothers, *Curanderas,* mother, will emphatically counsel their daughters to cover the heads of babies since they're believed to be conduits of illnesses.

Most cultures once believed in the need for balance in the bodily systems and that a lack of balance actually triggers sickness. A balance of hot and cold along with wet and dry should be strictly observed and maintained.

Anything that upsets the balance of these four factors will cause a dreaded illness.

LOST VALUABLES
AYÚDAME SAN ANTONIO

I am writing to you because I have lost my mother's cross that was on a necklace given to me by my father. It was passed on to me by my mother while she lay on her death bed. I am so scared I've lost it that if I can have it returned to me, I will never take it off again. I am so worried that I won't find it again. Can you please help me to find my necklace? Use the spirit world and the saints to help bring it back to me.

I do not know where your necklace is, but Saint Anthony does and he can help you find it. Try lighting a Saint Anthony candle. Make a promise to Saint Anthony that if he finds it and brings it back to you, you will do something for him like visit his shrine or offer a novena to him for the redemption of lost souls.

Once you promise, he will most likely place it in your path where you will find it.

Hispanic Curanderismo is inextricably intertwined with Roman Catholicism and its saints, beliefs and rituals. Saint Anthony is the patron saint of lost and misplaced items and as in Catholicism, *Curanderismo* recommends that prayer to Saint Anthony will be rewarded by the return of the lost item.

CLEAN YOUR HOUSE
EL DESPOJO

My grandmother would like to know if you can come to her house to cleanse it of evil forces and spirits. I know that you have a ritual for completely cleaning up a home from bad spirits and evil influences.

She wanted to visit you this week, but she's still having pain in her legs. Yesterday, she did so well that it seemed like the pain was going to go away for good. She had even slept a lot better than most nights.

She was so happy that she put the bedspreads on her beds and washed clothes like before she got this pain nearly four weeks ago. But, then, last night a little after midnight, she started complaining about the pain again and she didn't get relief until early this morning. She says that sometimes she gets relief after she cries.

Today she started drinking the *zacate de Limón* tea with *cenizo*. I see that *cenizo* is called sage and that *salvia* is also called sage.

I thank grandma for her faith and trust in my prayers. There are many deserving needs and requests for my efforts and services. I am honored she and you would have me cleanse her house.

Prepare a tea made from Lemon grass, *zacate de limón,* and *salvia,* not *cenizo,* for the pain.

Every Friday, burn incenses to the four winds and ask that the winds carry far away any and all negative forces that have attached themselves to your home during the week.

Medicinal plants are sometimes confused and called by inappropriate names. Sometimes plants have duplicate names in other geographical regions and there are variations of plants with similar names. One must always take care to have the proper plant because the wrong plant may produce undesirable effects or be no help at all.

Be sure to get real *salvia* and not sage. *Salvia* is the universal name for all sages in that particular plant family, but many varieties of sage are toxic. The correct *salvia* will be sold by any credible *hierbería, botánica,* herbalist, or Mexican products store.

HEXED
MALDICIÓN FAMILIAR

The first time I made this request, grandmother asked me to get two candles: a just judge, justo *juez* and Saint Gabriel, or seven Archangels' candle, for my happiness. The just judge candle would not stay lit. Each time I took out wax to find the wick, but it barely lit. I could only find the Saint Gabriel candle, which stays lit all the time. Last week, I was told to throw the candle away and get a new one.

I did, but the new one does the same thing. It has the dimmest light and does not seem to want to stay lit. I know that is not good. I am bathing in Holy Water and placing incense on the altar, as I was told for seven consecutive Fridays. The two new candles I got, always stay lit so I feel I'm on the right path now.

There is this guy that I really like, but he does not seem to care about me. Is something wrong with me? Some say that we have a family curse. Will you pray about it? I feel like this guy is playing with my emotions. He can be nice and then one minute later, he is heartless. He told me that he loved me, but now he acts as if he can't stand me. I don't understand. Does he really like me or should I just forget about him altogether? These are the things that I have been praying about.

It is difficult when you do not speak Spanish, the spirit will speak to your heart in the spiritual language and for that, you need no earthly language. Being in a spiritual trance helps us to communicate the union of the anointing and the giving and receiving of blessings.

The spirit advised you to burn the just judge, or *justo juez*, candles whenever possible. With your faith and prayer petitions, the doors to finding true love and true happiness shall be flung open for you. If this man is not your true soulmate, you will find someone who will truly love you for who you are. I am picking up that he has deep emotional problems and a history of doing to other women what he is doing to you.

There is nothing wrong with you. It seems to me there is something wrong with him! Do not give up and you will soon find your true love. You were advised to light the just judge candle for your petition so that the spirit could intercede and be your lawyer before God and plead on your behalf. You want to seek the happiness of the petitions you have made for true love in the form of an earthly companion in life.

Bathing with Holy Water and burning incense is for cleansing the person of negative energies, forces and influences. There is a big difference between liking somebody and being in love with someone. You know he is not in love with you so I feel it is time to let him go. I believe that if he was meant to be with you, he will return to you.

Hexes are routine in *Curanderismo.* Curses result from spells which have been cast by witches or *brujas* on people on behalf of other people. In Spanish, spells cast by witchcraft are called "works," or *trabajos. Curanderas* and *brujas* are known to conduct ongoing spell-casting and spell-breaking in a continual spiritual tug of war.

These mystical battles can last for decades and their *manda,* or cargo, can even be passed on to the next generation. Children and grandchildren continue a war of the witches and warlocks that they had nothing to do with from past generations.

USEFULL PSALMS
LOS SALMOS SANAN

Grandmother, I hear a lot about the power of the Psalms. I am a Catholic and we pray the Psalms. My mother, your daughter, is now a born-again Christian and they really pray the Psalms. In my limited experience with *Curanderas,* I have noticed that they almost always use the Psalms in their healing rituals. Should I be reading and praying the Psalms for my situations in life?

I am a healer and considered by some to possess *el don,* the spiritual gift of healing. My efforts are mainly concentrated to accompany those with health issues and in comforting and consoling them when I am asked to do so. I am a firm believer in the magical ability of the Psalms as handed down by King Solomon and King David, which is, *El Rey Salomón* and *El Rey David.*

In my altar room I have both the Holy Bible and the little book called the *Secrets of the Psalms.* I use them constantly. I read them during healings and you should do the same.

For example, in *Curanderismo,* a lot of my work is reversing bad luck and attracting good luck, but this is not a guarantee when it comes to wealth, money or winning the lottery. Divine Providence is always in the hands of God.

Many people try cleansings with heads of garlic and many other items to remove evil forces, spells, curses and bad luck, while others try spiritual healing baths to remove negative energies. Any method can work for you. It's all up to God.

Any one of Psalms 4, 8, 41, 43, 57, 61 and 63 may be used to return good luck or fortune to the household or to your business. If you need better luck or help with prosperity, then prepare an amulet bag of green flannel and place in the amulet bag black and yellow mustard seeds, a male garlic head, a copper coin, red and white coral, buckeye seed, juniper berry, and a whole spice and clove. Add a hot pepper, three coriander seeds and Irish moss leaves, two rose petals and horehound root. Mexican marketplaces sell these items as well as printed prayers for good luck and money drawing.

Personally, my favorite spell is to use essence of basil and seven male billy goat lotion, *loción siete machos*, for money-drawing purposes. Good luck and I hope you are granted all your wishes.

Most *Curanderas* perform simple white magic rites as spiritual trappings in their repertoires. *Curanderismo* is not just about healing, it also encompasses magic; this is why churches are mainly opposed to it.

Traditional *Curanderismo* is not self-serving. It is about helping the needy both materially and spiritually.

Curanderas habitually use spells to reverse a straying husband's ways, but spells used for personal gain are believed to lead to negative consequences. As *curandero*, *Don Perfecto* used to say, not only will you lose your spiritual power, but the spells you cast on others will come back on you. It's not worth it.

The Book of Psalms in the Old Testament, is believed to be handed down to us by King Solomon and King David, and is critically important in *Curanderismo*. The pamphlet entitled "Secrets of the Psalms" by Godfread Selig is readily available in *hierberías* and is considered an essential part of the *Curandera's* medicine bag. This little book addresses all nuances of life issues like court cases, escaping danger, how to receive holy blessings and many more.

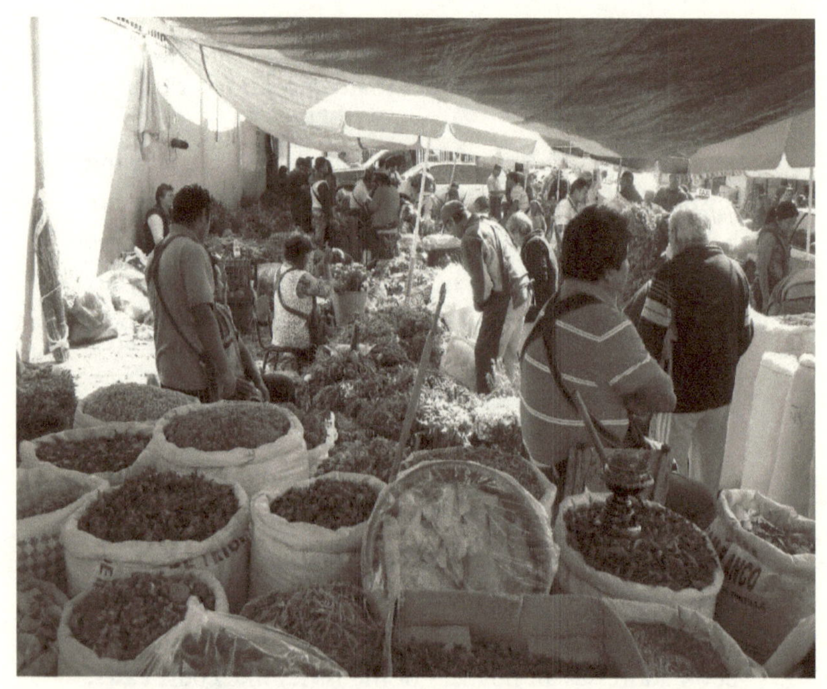

Open medicinal plant market, El Mercado Sonora

Part 3
Remedies for Romance and Betrayal

I AM ABANDONED
LA ABANDONADA

Purchase these four candles: *San Ignacio de Loyola*, *San Alejo*, a *San Cipriano* and a plain white candle for *San Eduardo*, the patron of good marriages and for *Saint Gummarus*, who is acknowledged on October 11, and is the patron of the unhappy marriages. All are seven-day candles. Once you have all four candles, or four plain white wax, seven-day candles, place them in a triangle. Position one on the east side where the sun rises and the other two on the west side where the sun sets. Place his picture in the center of the three candles. Place the fourth candle in the center along with a clear glass of water over his photo.

Light the candles and make your petition to the Lord asking to have your husband return home. Once you light the candles, do not extinguish them. This candle-burning ritual is to clear him of all the witchcraft influences that have been placed on him by the other woman or by anyone else. This should work within about seven to nine days.

It is common in *Hispanic* culture to use magical spells performed by practitioners known as *brujas* or witches to draw people into sexual relationships or to break up relationships. More than likely, this is what the other woman has done to your husband.

While it may sound very strange or foreign to those who have not heard of this, it is actually one of the most routine requests made of healers and witches, *Curanderas* and *brujas*.

The witch is asked to destroy a marriage and the *Curandera* is asked to return the husband to his rightful wife. The *Curandera* intimates to the wife that this is why her husband is afraid of her and stays away from his daughter, family and friends.

This strange behavior can only be understood within the context of witchcraft. This is supported by his inability to go anywhere alone except to work.

DESTROYED MARRIAGE
BRUJERÍA DESTRUYE MATRIMONIO

Grandmother, I have been going through some very troubling times. My husband has been seeing another woman, but recently and with your help, my husband has broken off with the woman that he thought was the love of his life. This illicit relationship was destroying my marriage and my children at the same time.

I have been feeling awkward the last couple of years and have found myself spiritually weakened at times. I went to see a psychic and this lady gave me a reading that was completely accurate. She also told me that someone went to an evil witch, or *bruja,* and asked this witch to cast a spell upon me and my marriage using the devil, pure evil.

This bad witch was paid a lot of money and agreed to cast the spell, called a *trabajo.* Together, my husband's girlfriend and the witch have brought misery, pain and suffering upon every aspect of my life.

I hired a witch to perform a ritual to reverse the spell. I think I wasted my time and my money. I was really very nervous about it because she asked me to bring $1,800 and I wasn't sure what it was being used for. She said that the money was needed to use against the warlock, or *bruja*, who laid out the curse on my marriage. She said she spent it all to destroy the spell against us. I don't know if this is true or not. This has been going on for a couple of years now.

The *bruja* also rubbed an egg on my body to pull out of me anything that was evil. During this ritual we broke the egg and I saw something in it that really scared me. I was in total disbelief. I saw the mark of a hand with a claw with blood and it looked like the devil's hand. That's what my *bruja* said it was.

My husband and I are caught in the devil's hand and the devil is squeezing the life out of our marriage.

The *bruja* then cut the $1,800 I gave her in half because she said the people that did this to me used the mark of the beast or 666 on me because they thought that I would not be able to raise this amount of money to reverse the spell. They used that same number to break the curse.

The *bruja* said that we had to cut up the money and mix it in with the egg. The *bruja* says that the evil is attempting to destroy my marriage so my husband will be under the eternal spell of his girlfriend.

What kind of woman would do this to a marriage with children? I was told that the number of the beast, 666, adds up to the number 18. So, the psychic has told me that $600 times 3 makes $1,800 which is the amount I would need to reverse the devil's number. The *bruja* says she has to complete the ritual and has asked that I call her back later to learn the results.

I now know that my husband's girlfriend also spent a lot of money to purchase the evil necessary to cover my eyes, *tapa ojos,* and take my husband away from me. I keep asking the *bruja* for the name of the person who has cursed me but she says that it is too dangerous to tell me the name right now until the spell is reversed.

But I think I know who it is. I just want her to say her name out loud so I can be satisfied I know. I know it was my husband's girlfriend because they told me at work it was. Her girlfriends are also terrified that she will take their men away.

Since I contacted you and you put me on the righteous path, I know that there is a spiritual battle taking place right now between me and my husband's girlfriend. The witch she is using is one of the most powerful in this area. People have even seen her shapeshift into an owl, or *lechuza.*

The *bruja* told me that she would go to church and complete the ritual in order to reverse or break this spell. She said that she had to burn my money and the egg and bury them in the church yard and then it would be finished. But I don't believe her. I think she just ripped me off. I threw my hard-earned money away. I don't want this evil on me. I want to walk the path of light, and I want my marriage put back together.

I ask you to give me the strength and will to live a good and healthy life. I ask you to show me the light and the right way to live. Show me how to love and restore my husband and to help my kids and most importantly, help my husband not to want to see his girlfriend again. I wish to know the truth.

Grandmother, I am very confused, and my mother and aunt asked me to consult you for guidance because you have helped them in the past. I do believe I need your help; this evil spell is too strong to defeat by myself.

You made a huge mistake giving the witch your money. Your problem will be solved with faith and prayer and the workers in the light; not with dirty money.

Secondly, I believe I can guide and help you in your situation. I will pray over you for your spiritual deliverance and healing.

To begin your spiritual cleansing and healing, light three white candles forming a triangle with the three candles, one on the east side and two to the west side, placing a picture of yourself in the center and a clear glass of water over your picture. You need to call out a saint's name three times and make your petition to him.

The saint's spirit will come to you and will begin to help you. Also, buy a green candle and dedicate it to *San Cipriano* who will also protect you from any kind of witchcraft that is affecting your marriage.

LOVE IS GONE
YA NO ME QUIERE

Grandmother, my husband has abandoned me and the kids. I don't know what to do or what's going on with him. Do you "see" another woman in his life? He has not given me any reason to think so. I have been taking my garlic baths but so far, I don't think they are working. The kids miss him a lot and I don't know what to tell them. I don't have the money to move. I thought we had a happy marriage. Can you see if there is something else that is bothering him? Help me to save my marriage?

The garlic baths are for spiritual cleansing and the ridding of evil curses, witchcraft spells, hexes and bad luck.

Place a pinch of cinnamon powder inside your shoes every morning when you get up then say a prayer. Cleanse yourself with a lemon while praying the Lord's Prayer, *El Padre Nuestro.*

Another thing you can do is purchase three yellow candles, and beginning on a Thursday, place his photo and your photo facing one another in front of one candle. Tie the photos together with yellow string always circling clockwise never counterclockwise. Place the photos and the candle on a yellow cloth and sweeten the item by either sprinkling a little sugar on it or dripping a little honey over it. Get a yellow rose and pull off the petals and place them around the candle and photos. Repeat the procedure for three weeks, always on Thursdays and always starting during the early morning hours. Start each week with a new candle, the same photos, but with a new yellow rose.

At the end of three weeks, dispose of all the materials you used in water in which the water current is running toward your home. This ritual will also serve to bring your husband home to his family.

One of the most popular reasons people seek advice from a *Curandera* is for marital or relationship issues. Not able to resolve personal problems themselves, these suffering individuals seek aid from the *Curandera* or resort to witchcraft to influence an errant loved one, morally guide a wayward spouse home or to extinguish the other woman's hold.

ADDICTIONS
VICIOSO

Grandmother wanted to give a woman who visited her a ritual cleansing or *limpia* but the older man, said that he did not believe in these things and refused. Grandmother said they could come back any time. The woman pleaded with her husband to get the cleansing and he agreed that she could get one if she wanted. He said he was an alcoholic and that the only reason he came was to please his wife.

I cut some fresh branches from the lavender shrub to use for the cleansing ritual, and the three of us went to grandmother's altar room to perform the healing ritual.

While we were there, I asked the man if he believed in God and he said that he did. I explained that during the cleansing ritual he could ask for a healing from God. I told him that I was there just to help him along. He looked into my eyes and he acknowledged once again he did believe in God. I lifted my hand to touch his forehead with the herbs, and as the herbs touched his forehead, he began to jerk frantically backward and forward. His legs were unable to support his weight, and as his wife tried to keep him from falling, he fell into a chair.

The ritual instantaneously brought about a terrible resistance in him and the prayers brought about an even greater torment from within the subject. Luckily, for me I was able to control him with her help. With a simple touch, something changed in him and he was no longer the same person. There seemed to be the appearance of another being in him.

I immediately could see that this other being was very angry and could possibly turn violent at any moment. As the anger built up, I was fearful and wanted to get away, but I had a job to do.

I began the healing ritual and it became an exorcism. He calmed down and appeared to become himself once again and acknowledged that he was an alcoholic, and that he used cocaine and marijuana on a regular basis. He said he would return for further healing.

In the old days, there was another way in which women would control their husbands' drinking. In the *hierbería* you can find *habas de San Ignacio,* a sort of round flat bean from a tree in Mexico. Women grind them up and mix them in their spouses' meals in small amounts to induce vomiting when they drink. Thus, it is believed that they would not want to drink.

Extensive research has been conducted on gender and cultural factors which influence drug and alcohol addiction as well as rehabilitation. There are many cultural methods which mimic current medical treatments for addiction.

For example, the *habas de San Ignacio* bean mentioned by the *Curandera* should be treated very carefully because it has been proven to induce vomiting. The same type of therapy that induces nausea is used in some medications and produces similar results. The person who is feeling nauseous does not feel like drinking.

Control of substance abuse must always be sustained by a combination of behavior modification with medication prescribed by a doctor.

Families with alcoholic relatives will often give them tea made from *estafiate,* or mugwort. Antihepatotoxins are medicinal plants believed to fortify the liver. An antidote, or *antídoto,* is the action of a plant used to reverse an action from another plant.

MAKING AMENDS
CONFORMÁNDOSE

Create your own very special prayer for a husband and wife and a happy life together. Pray together before retiring for the day. If the other is absent, pray alone, but for the intentions of the couple. Pray something like this:

"Santa Ana, we pray to you to continue to bless us, help us to appreciate you for what we have. We are united by the sacrament of matrimony. Grant that we will truly be one in heart and mind, and that we respect each other's person. Grant that we love one another, remembering it was you who gave us our love because we should be parents to your children. Help us to give one another completely and be less egotistical and trust one another. Help us to trust our difficulties in you and to always count on the promise that you gave us in the sacrament of matrimony. Help us to be good parents to our family. Be it your will to grant us health and the strength for our duties in the happiness that supports us in our love. Grant that we not forget that we have been given a blessing from heaven by the grace of our Lord and Savior. God give us strength, valor and blessing so that it may go well through our journey. Amen."

Also, it is a good idea to maintain a specially-prepared candle lighted at noon every day for 21 straight days. Be sure to write both of your names in red ink on a piece of paper and place the candle over it while it is burning.

Some spells for repairing broken marriages or relationships use the root and the seed of *High John the Conqueror, Raiz de Juan el Conquistador*. Then write the name of the man on the root and the name of the woman on the seed, sprinkle them with perfume and place them in a small red cloth bag. The bag is then carried on your person, either in a pocket or pinned to inner clothing.

Grandmother composed a very special spiritual prayer in this case. The petitioner asked for and received the specially-requested prayer to save her marriage. She also received a vital healing regimen which included her husband's participation. Praying together can show the spouse a form of rededication to God and the marriage.

WE NEED SPIRITUAL HELP
NO NOS AYUDA

Grandmother, says my child, I know you are going through a lot and my prayers are with you. Do a cleansing/healing with a lemon for nine consecutive days. Don't throw the lemons away. Say a prayer to the *Virgen* that unties knots, her name is *Santa María de Desatanudos,* and make your petition while doing the cleansing.

At the end of the nine *limpias*, make a fire and burn the nine lemons you used for the nine days of cleansings.

Grandmother does not address the reason that the husband has emotionally abandoned his family. In all likelihood, he has his own problems and is not able to provide support for his family, especially his son. There could be another woman or another family involved here, we simply don't know. He may also be ashamed of his son and blames his wife for the son's problems, refusing to be accountable for his own parental role and responsibilities.

Often, the personal issues of husbands and wives are interwoven, further complicating familial issues. I can see you talking to your daughter, providing her with advice, but you need to keep your life out of it or she won't listen to you. After all, she knows your history as well as you do. She will think that you are trying to meddle in her life, and you are.

She is confused and being pulled in different directions. She does not know which way to go. She needs to see what would be best for her happiness and most importantly, for her baby's welfare. She needs you to be there helping her find a solution, but don't be overpowering.

You should advise your daughter not to make hasty decisions. She should not rush into any relationship. Her whimsical behavior is what got her into serious problems in the first place. You and your daughter should place your daughter's child's welfare first and foremost before making any decisions around that issue.

Whatever you do, do not use her father as a bad example you throw at her. That will surely backfire and turn your daughter against you.

I am sure you are keeping her in your prayers. Please, light a candle, or a Saint Michael the Archangel candle for your daughter. Place a glass of water by the candles and say a prayer. She will help the true couple that is meant to be together.

The close-knit nature of the *Hispanic* family produces situations where everyone is very connected in each other's lives and decisions, both good and bad. In this case, it is quite obvious that the mother is very meddlesome in her daughter's life.

The mother's life is possibly not much better than her daughter. The mother has committed so many mistakes that she's now living vicariously through her daughter's situation. The generational differences between the mother and daughter further exacerbate their problems.

This projection of the same fate is both unhealthy and inappropriate behavior. The only thing that counts here is the welfare of the child. What the daughter and the mother want are not as important. The mother must set aside her life and experiences so that the daughter and granddaughter can prosper.

LIFE'S DILEMAS
DILEMAS DE LA VIDA

Grandmother, I understand what you are telling me. Light a *Sagrado Corazón,* Sacred Heart of Jesus, candle for peace. Cleanse everyone in the household with a *San Alejo* and a *San Ignacio de Loyola* candle. Use the same ones for all the family. Put a pinch of cinnamon powder, a pinch of sugar, a few mustard seeds and a few rosemary leaves inside the candles.

Place a clear glass of water over the pictures of everyone in the family next to the candles. Light the candles and make your petitions to the Holy Spirit.

Boil rosemary in the evenings and make your petition to God for light, understanding, love, happiness and peace. Do this for nine consecutive nights.

The garlic baths are for spiritual cleansing from evil, curses, witchcraft spells, hexes and bad luck. Place a pinch of cinnamon powder inside your shoes every morning when you get up to start your day and pray to

San Eduardo, saying "Follow in my footsteps and answer my prayers this day, oh, *San Eduardo.* Favor me before the eyes of my fellow man, oh, *San Eduardo.*" Cleanse yourself with a lemon and pray the Lord's Prayer.

Purchase a magnet stone, or *piedra imán,* from the nearest *hierbería,* along with nine white candles and oil for peace and calm as well as *conquistador,* or conqueror oil. Place three white candles in a triangle with the *piedra imán,* magnet stone, in the middle for three weeks always beginning Thursday. Be sure that you drip or spray the two essences of peace oil and *conquistado*r oil over the area.

Write your name and your husband's name on parchment paper and also place this in the middle of the three candles. You will see your husband begin to change his attitude toward you.

Many Hispanics find themselves in despairing situations. They are trapped in marriages without love, but with children who depend upon them. They are culturally bound to stay in their marriages despite being miserable. This causes behavioral health issues that need an outlet. Persons in great need of an emotional safety valve often find solace in a sympathetic healer.

The informal networks of friends they encounter at the *Curandera's* spiritual healing sessions are similar to a 12-step program. While waiting to be seen by the *Curandera,* much is discussed and learned from the people awaiting their turns at consultation.

I NEED SOMEONE IN MY LIFE
ALGUIEN PARA MÍ

This is for my special friends who are in love, but never seem to spend time together. The person, who finds love, peace and happiness in himself, has these same qualities to share with others. To remove these barriers and clear the way, or *abre camino*, the spirit indicates you may place seven *pencas de nopal*, or cactus leaves, in a bucket of water and set the bucket out in the daylight for seven consecutive hours. Most importantly, call upon *San Antonio* to protect the lovers in this case. Then petition that the obstacles to your love be removed from your path.

To remove obstacles from her way place seven *tunas*, or prickly pear fruit, in a pail of water left in daylight for seven hours, and thereafter bathe with the water. The leaves and the fruit of the cactus are the male and female elements of the common Mexican cactus, or *nopal*.

It is also possible to bind up love with a red ribbon saturated with special love potions or perfumes. Write your loved one's name on the red ribbon at high noon on a Friday, then, apply the perfume. While you do this, always concentrate on the name of the person and visualize their face. Pin the ribbon inside your inner garments for 21 consecutive days.

The grandmother offers a classic love-attraction ritual intended to draw the lovers together. Incantations designed to attract or inspire the affection of another were practiced within European as well as in Mesoamerican magical rites.

Over the centuries, methodology has evolved, but always retained the intent of using magical means to transform outcomes of romantic attractions. In the world of today's *Curanderas,* the practice uses all of the modern paraphernalia found in the *hierbería* for this purpose.

This includes sprays, wax figures, powders, oils, soaps, perfumes and much more. There are many ways to do this and no single or absolute method.

The grandmother uses an element of sympathetic magic in the male and-female aspects of the same cactus plant in a ritual to consummate the relationship. One of the most frequently consulted books in the hierbería is the book of *San Cipriano.*

This little grimorio, or book of magic, claims to have been compiled in the year 1001, by *Jonas Sufurino* a monk who studied mysticism and magic. Today, *San Cipriano* is considered the patron saint of magicians and is believed to protect them against spells, demons and evil in general. The book contains many commonly-used spells, or sortilegios, regarding marriage, relationships and love affairs.

For example: How to fall in love; how to discover if a woman is seeing another man; how to know if a husband is faithful, and many other romantic spells are contained in this mystical tome. Sex, love, and relationships are among the most requested categories that *Curanderas* deal with on a daily basis.

THE WRONG MAN
EL TONTO

Grandmother, I had trouble with a guy and I'm still having trouble with him. I met him and fell in love with him. Then, all of a sudden, he stopped calling me. Now I have no contact with him at all.

I am writing to you again because I don't know what is going on. I find myself constantly thinking about this man. It is like a feeling you get when someone is talking about you, a very strong feeling. I tried forgetting about him, but it didn't work. I still like him and that is not all.

There's another guy I know and I don't understand why I think about him all the time, too. He comes and goes out of my mind and I don't know what's going on. I don't understand why I have all these desires. He seems like a nice guy and I like him a lot, but I haven't seen him since we were teenagers.

Back then we were never given an opportunity to have a relationship. Please help me out and let me know what's going on in my head and in my heart. I would like to get married and have children someday. I'm still single and am lonely.

Has someone put a spell on me so I can't fall in love and have a normal relationship?

If the guy is not meant to be the love of your life you should try to forget him and move on. I am sure there is someone out there that will fall madly in love with you and you with him. Please try my spiritual healing advice. You shall see what I am talking about.

Light a candle to Saint Gabriel the Archangel and make your petition for happiness in life. If you do not find that candle, look for the seven archangels' candle and boil *gobernadora, alhucema,* cinnamon sticks, four, cut apples and rose petals with a cup of honey and bathe in this water at noon on Friday while saying a prayer to Saint Gabriel Archangel.

Single Hispanics are under a constant psychological cultural barrage from their own families and friends to enter into a relationship leading to marriage and a family.

As more year's pass, those still not engaged begin to feel a gradual buildup of familial pressure and a sense of personal failure. This *tía*, or aunt syndrome requires them to take on the role of the surrogate mother to their nephews and nieces. But they go unfilled as wives and mothers in life.

BANISH MY RIVAL
LÍBRAME

Grandmother, my ex-boyfriend has missed two days of work due to a woman he is messing around with. He told me yesterday that he is probably going to have to move back with my son and me because this woman refuses to leave his apartment.

Now she is threatening that she will go to his probation officer to tell him he's been doing drugs if he leaves her. She is telling him that she has pictures of them doing drugs which she plans to tell his probation officer. This evil woman is holding him hostage from his past. I guess the hold that she has on him is sex and drugs.

I always thought that he wanted to live a decent family life, but I'm no longer certain. I am still praying and I have lit some candles. I do not understand why this woman is being so difficult and will not leave.

I don't believe that the two of you are compatible. Why can't you see that he is no good? Your relationship may never improve. You are having problems admitting that you are not right for each other. It may be time for you to do the right thing for yourself and accept change. Move on with your life. Expect powerful and positive changes for yourself.

Also, bathe in a bath prepared with rosemary, mint, anise, star anise, basil and myrrh and add High John the Conqueror seed.

One-way women may control their men is through the use of jimson weed, or *toloache*. If she is truly evil, this is what she is using. Jimson weed is a powerful herb and, in small amounts, it's used to control men and women and to settle them down to stay home and not fool around. Usually, they don't know that they are being given the substance, which keeps them docile, or *mansitos*.

We simply do not know what has transpired between the woman and the *Curandera*. It seems like the *Curandera* has not offered hope, only an easy exit. The ex-boyfriend is vain and maybe he just wants to come home and feel loved.

The *Curandera* psychically "sees" the truth and sometimes there is no hope for the relationship to survive. The *Curandera* tells the woman about jimson weed, also known as *toloache*.

This is a *datura,* and Mexican populations have used it for centuries to control straying husbands. It has a very powerful effect and should not be used by someone who is not fully versed in how to properly prepare and dispense it.

THE DIVORCE
EL DIVORCIO

Grandmother, my wife has asked me for a divorce and we have a seven-month-old baby boy. I really love my son and I will do anything for him. I am very confused about why my wife is doing this to our family.

My wife and I had an apartment so we split up and I moved to my sister's house and my wife moved to her friend's house. She told me yesterday that after living with her friend, she realized that her mom was the real reason she was mad at me all the time because her mom would tell her how to be a good wife to me and she would get upset and, in turn, get mad at me. This has been going on since she got pregnant and finally, she decided that she had enough and wanted a divorce.

After causing all of this confusion in our lives, now she tells me that she would like to try and work things out. She would like to get an apartment and live away from her mom instead of living in our house, which is being built next to her mom's. She says she would like for us to live on our own so she can have a chance to grow up without being in her mom's shadow.

I told her that I would also like to work things out and that we could get the apartment and sell the house. I told her that she and her mom had to get counseling to deal with their problems. She is very quiet and never wants to talk about her problems, and avoids confrontation and holds everything in until she finally blows up. She agreed to get some help and also take her mom to get some help.

I am willing to try and make our marriage work so we can be a united family and my child can grow up in a complete family instead of a broken home.

Grandmother, can you ask the spirits if moving in with her and working things out is the right thing to do, or if she is just setting me up?

I have been keeping you in my prayers for some time now. Regarding your situation now is not the time to rush into anything. Take your time about getting back together until you are sure she is not setting you up for anything nor has a hidden motive.

When your wife is sure she is ready to settle down and be a responsible mother to your child and a wife, you will know it. When she is convinced that she is ready and can convince you of it, then it will be time to make the marriage work, not before.

Divorce can truly be one of the most traumatic and bitter events individuals experience in their lives. Persons should not have to go through a divorce without a support network.

In the *Hispanic* culture, grandmothers and *Curanderas* play major roles in the familial support network. If you decide to consult a *Curandera* for delicate issues like this one, you must find a reputable person to assist you.

MY RIVAL
MI RIVAL

Grandmother, I am writing you in regards to my mother. She wants your prayers and any advice you can give her. The woman that my father had an affair with is making it as hard as she possibly can for my mother.

First of all, this woman filed a restraining order against my mother, but my mother is the one that is severely hurt in all this mess.

Then, this woman keeps trying to get a hold of my father by calling our home, knowing all along that my mother is bound by the terms of the restraining order she placed against her. There is not much she can do.

To make matters worse, my father refuses to answer my mother's calls and now my mother has been fired from her job. My mother worked at the same place with this other woman, but my mother is the one that got fired.

This other woman has been trying to get my mom in trouble for any little thing she can. If my mother goes anywhere, she has to be looking over her shoulder because if the other woman sees her, she calls the police. The woman tells the police that my mother is following her, but of course this is not true.

My mother and aunt were out recently and were walking out of a store and they saw the woman and her mother. My father's girlfriend's mom pointed out my mom and my aunt, and the woman created a huge scandal by yelling at my mom that she was going to call the cops. She got on her cell phone and called.

My mom left before she could finish the call, but the cops showed up at my mom's home and told her that the next time, they will take my mom to jail. The officers told my mom that there is a stack of complaint forms at the police station against her.

Then, as if that was not bad enough, my mom has received a letter with a court date accusing her of violating the restraining order. She spoke to a lawyer today to represent her. It will cost her over a $1,000 to defend herself and the lawyer said if anyone should have a restraining order against anyone it should be my mom against the other woman, and I agree. My mother never asked for any of this. She is very worried about her court date.

Grandmother, please pray for her so that she will have a just judge, *justo juez*. My mom wishes that the woman would just leave this town forever. I wish she would just leave my mother and my father alone. Why can't she find her own man, why does she have to have my father? I hope that in court the other woman can feel the shame and embarrassment my mom has been feeling.

Pray to *San Cipriano* for all your family. Burn some candles for your mom's safety, protection and well-being. Tell your mom to call grandmother and, if your mom could, have her go to a *hierbería* and purchase a *San Alejo* and a *San Ignacio de Loyola's* even-day candle. When she does that, she can call me and I will explain how she will use them to get rid her of all the problems this woman has created for her.

Some persons know how to manipulate the system, but they are definitely on the other side of righteousness. Frequently, they use the police and courts for selfish and harmful gains. The wife needs an authority figure to serve as her advocate.

There must be someone who knows the reputation of the other woman or her work situation who can help or testify against her. It appears this other woman has done this before. The mother should enlist her personal network of family and friends to resolve this troublesome issue.

Notice that this is a perfect example of a case that could include the use of witchcraft to manipulate the situation, but it wasn't mentioned by the petitioner or by the *Curandera*.

RETURN HIM TO ME
VEN A MÍ

Grandmother, I followed your instructions and the candles are now burning. They should burn out in seven days. What do I do next to get my husband to return to me? I have been praying and believing in God for his return. Please let me know what I need to do next.

Pray to Saint Gabriel the Archangel and to *San Daniel*, then, make your petition. Place a clear glass of water on your kitchen table or on your home altar. Call out the name of the archangel aloud three times and repeat the prayer. Do this for nine consecutive days.

Light a just judge, or *justo juez*, candle, and another plain white candle. Get romance and attracting perfumes or sprays named, come to me, or *ven a mí*, from the *hierbería*. Place them or spray them on your left hand and place your left hand over your heart. Pray for your man to return.

If your relationship is growing cold you need a ritual that will sweeten it. That is to bring back the passion. A qualified Curandera will be required to perform the ritual of sweetening your relationship.

Candle-burning rituals are universal in the practice of magic around the world. The Catholic priests introduced candle burning to Latin American populations in the 16th century. The dark side of witchcraft is thought to reverse Catholic rituals. Therefore, candle burning is common in the practice of both white and black magic. Black magic is used to darken good which is opposite of the original intent of illuminating our prayers with candles.

THE CHEATING HUSBAND
EL ENGAÑO

I have been married for years and now my husband has left me. We have grown children. He went to truck-driving school, and soon after went out on the road. Not long after that, he met a woman who is also a truck driver and they started a relationship. Now they are driving a truck together. In the last six months, he has gone from being a loving family man to no longer caring about neither being home nor seeing his family. Can you please tell me if you can help me to get my husband back?

You have a serious dilemma if your husband abandoned his family for another woman. If he is unfaithful to you this time, how can you be sure that you would have a good marriage if he were to return to you?

What is to keep him from doing the same thing again and again? I would suggest that you start anew. Do not ask someone to do witchcraft to get him back.

Curanderas use multiple time-tested means to work with wayward spouses and their lovers. First, illnesses that are attributed to all three of those involved, are believed to have natural origins. God and the saints find the situation morally repugnant and mete out punishment through sickness.

At one time, *Curanderas* would recommend the herb *toloache,* or *datura* for wayward husbands to keep *them docile, or toloachado.* This dangerous herb would literally render them physically unable to leave their homes, or keep them *mansos.*

You may have noticed from this series of spousal relationships, that partners stray when the relationship becomes mundane and new persons enter the lives of one or both of the marital partners. This is why it is always important for couples to maintain communication and be open with each other.

Like a beautiful garden, marriages also need constant tending for successful growth. This care could manifest via a date night without the kids, a weekend getaway, and notes of affection or even romantic poems for emotional sustenance.

MY WIFE HAS A LOVER
EL OTRO

Grandmother, I want to ask you about the candles you asked me to buy to get rid of all negative forces and bring my wife back to me. I found out this man she is seeing has my picture buried inside a glass jar somewhere in my yard. A family member told me about this, and that I need to be careful because the man is trying to steal my woman away from me and maybe even kill me.

I have talked to my former wife and she feels that some force is keeping her in the other man's house and won't let her leave. When she tries to come to my house, something pulls her back. She told me she wants to leave him and that if she has to, she will move out. But when she mentions this to him, he flies into a rage and says that his *bruja,* or witch, will kill her if she leaves him. So, she is afraid to leave him.

This is a clear sign of witchcraft. Please let me know what to do. My prayers are with you, and you are not alone. The spirit of *San Valentín* is with you. He is a healing spirit of light, a spirit guide, a spirit protector, a spirit doctor, a spirit lawyer, a spirit counselor. His spirit will help you. His spirit will place medicine in your body, mind and soul. This spiritual medicine will give you strength, valor, and the will to overcome any witchcraft that has been placed on you.

Make yourself a red stone amulet bag. Obtain a small red felt bag or make one and place a red stone signifying the heart inside the bag. Sometimes, you can find small red hearts which would be perfect.

Apply love and attraction perfumes on the stone then carry it with you.

Since the practice of witchcraft is so widespread, it is understandable that persons who do not partake in witchcraft encounter mystical items without even realizing what they are.

Never touch these items with your bare hands! When in doubt, always contact a competent healer who is experienced in destroying these objects in the proper manner, which is usually by fire.

STAY AWAY
DÉJALO IR

Grandmother, so much has happened and I have been trying to cope with my depression. Just last week I wanted to take my life, but I asked God for strength.

My heart is heavy because of that woman who lives in my ex-husband's home. He threw her out once and we started to work things out and planned to move back together. Things were going great until she started writing to him again and then he took her back.

Last week he was so ugly to our son and me. Someone sent the police to my job, and claimed that I broke into his house. That is a lie! Someone broke into my home and took a lot of things from me. I have a chance to file charges against them, but I am torn because I love him. My son is also deeply disturbed. Do you see any chance for our relationship? Do you see him in my picture anymore or is he gone for good? I really need your advice now as I have no one to turn to.

Grandmother, everything in my life had started to change for the good and suddenly things have turned ugly again. Please tell me if there is anything good coming my way in the future or are things just going to get worse?

Is my ex-husband going to be a part of my son's life even if we are not together? He has been the only father my son has known since he was three years old and he is now 17.

You may need to let him go for your welfare and your son's. Your son is old enough now to understand. He received the benefit of a father for all those years. You had a man, but if he cheated one time, he will do it again. I don't think he will change back to the man you once knew.

It may be time for you to turn the page and start a new life. You might be asking God for something that is not good for you in which case He will not grant it.

Ask *Santa María Desatanudos* to "untie the knots" that bind you and to give you strength to go on with your son and your life. Your life and your intentions are pure, love will come to you again when you least expect it.

False accusations, accompanied by robbery and lying to the police, are obvious and very disturbing warning signs. Suppressed rage and domestic problems always lead to violence. Try, at all costs, to avoid situations that may lead to domestic violence before a family problem escalates into serious legal problems.

RID ME OF THIS WOMAN
QUÍTAMELA

Grandmother, help me get rid of the woman those lives with me. This woman, together with her mother and her children, does me much more harm than good. I'm so depressed about all of the many dreadful things they do to me.

I don't know why I put up with it, a force of habit I suppose. They are not happy and don't appreciate that I'm providing housing, education, and supporting them, despite them not being my children.

They pay me back by making fun of me, screaming and humiliating me. They do not value anything I do for them. She drinks a lot and gets home late. I don't know where she has been and I put up with it because I don't want to live by myself again. I am afraid to be alone and that is why I put up with this.

Yes, of course I will help you. But you must want to help yourself first! Prepare a crystal glass with water and keep it in the middle of your kitchen table. Every time the woman leaves the house, without her knowing what you are doing, throw the water from the glass toward her back on the floor or outside just after she walks out.

Also, have a regular household broom and position the bottom side up and behind the front door of the house. At every opportunity, when she leaves the house, sweep behind her and out the door. Whatever you do, don't let her see what you are doing. This is in order to avoid her becoming angry; because then the one who'll be running out is you. Do all this with caution and everything will work out.

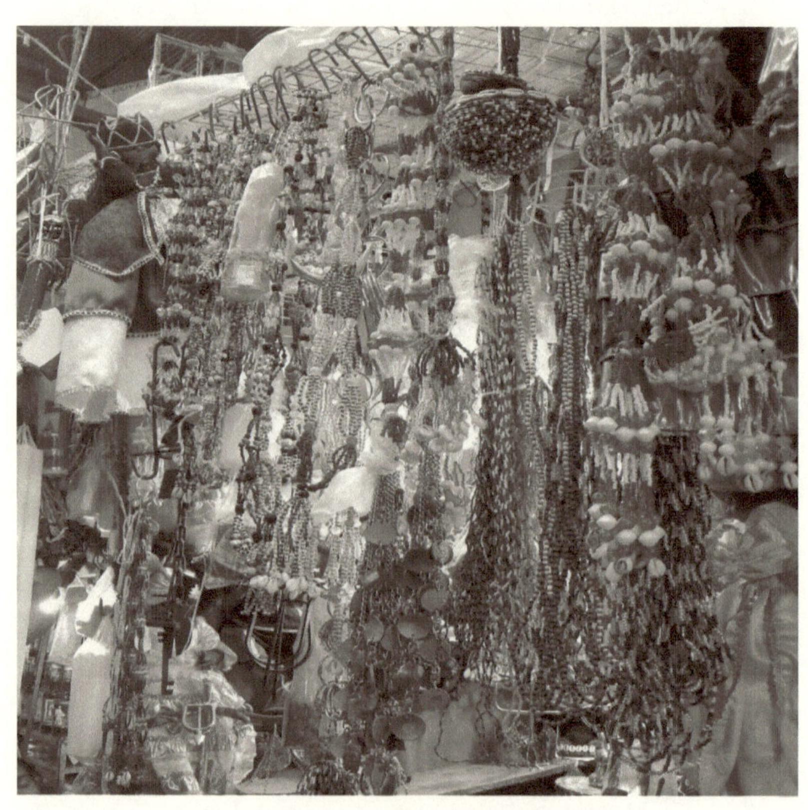

Santeria Beads at The Mercado Sonora

Part 4
Remedies for Justice

WIN COURT CASE
JUSTO JUEZ

Grandmother, is there a certain candle that is used to influence the outcome of court cases? I know that there is and that it is blue. What I don't understand is does the glass have to be blue, the wax or both?

I want to win my divorce case; I was told to put my husband's picture under the candle and to have a plain glass of water next to the candle.

Yes, there is a specially-made candle for petitions for legal matters and court cases and it comes in a blue wax. You may use a plain, blue wax candle if you do not find the original. You may also elect to use a *Saint Jude* candle, the patron saint for impossible causes and a *justo juez,* or just judge, candle.

Saint *Joan of Arc* may always be invoked to protect the powerless against the powerful. Her day of celebration is on May 30. Either one will work.

Pray Psalms 38 and 39 to protect those who are being punished by the law. Importantly, the correct candle for a court case is always in blue wax. Yes, place the glass of water over your husband's picture next to the candle you have lit.

The use of *justo juez* and *law-stay-away* candles has become increasingly popular in the *Hispanic* community. Additionally, powders, oils, sprays and other items are believed to be spiritually effective in legal cases. As an unfortunate side note, *La Santísima Muerte, Malverde, Pancho Villa* and other entities are commonly used to influence the law and legal cases. They are not bad, by themselves, but are frequently used by people who commit crimes. Attempting to influence outcomes of court cases has become a common exercise among law-abiding citizens as well as scofflaws.

DRUGS KILL
DROGAS MATAN

Grandmother, I wrote to you before and am writing again in regards to my out of-control life! I have been smoking marijuana for a long time and I have used other kinds of drugs as well. I was in a yearlong abusive relationship and have been in jail many times and I am finally ready to go straight.

I prayed last night for the first time in a long time. I left my boyfriend and all my friends to free myself from the pressure to do drugs. I do not want to be close to them.

I am scared because I am still in trouble with the cops, the court and probation. I am ready to clean up my life and serve God, for once and all. I want to confess all of my sins and start over.

I regret and hate the things I have done in my life. I am a very smart girl who the Lord has blessed with many talents. I do not want to go to jail again. I no longer want any drugs in my body. I am ready to start over without my old boyfriend coming around.

I do not want to be weak and give in to the pressure of drugs. I want a new life and I want to be finally out of trouble!

Please, is there anything I can do to get my body clean of these drugs, other than giving it time? Are there any prayers you can send me to help me? Most of all, please pray for me!

Pray to the Holy Spirit to help you to turn away from those who disobey Him. It is good that you have repented from evil and your wicked ways. It is good that you want to turn your back on disobedience and turn to the Lord's ways.

Pray to *Saint Maximilian Kolbe* that you abandon a life of drugs and I pray that the Lord will answer your prayers and bestow His blessings in abundance upon you. Are you ready to take the high road in your life?

Allow your spirit to be your guide. You have reached a critical fork in the road of your life. It has become clear to your which path to take.

The journey through life can be what you are willing to make it. The best in life will not come easy. It will take hard work to get you to where you want to be. If you live your convictions, it will help you live a happy and full life. The Holy Spirit will help you through hard times.

If you truly are ready to confess you must do it out loud and pray to Saint Pio the patron of confession to hear your confession and to absolve you of your sins.

As in all populations, many *Hispanics* suffer from a combination of physical and emotional issues; exacerbated by social and cultural nuances. Often, these individuals are unable to access professional counseling, so they turn to culturally-based systems like *Curanderismo*. Additionally, they feel more at ease talking to someone from their own culture.

WINNING THE CASE
GANANDO LA CAUSA

Grandmother, I'm writing to you for my mother. She wants me to ask you to pray for her upcoming court date. A while back, she was injured on the job. Her back has been hurt very badly since then. She is trying to get restitution due to her for her loss of wages.

The corporate lawyers are going against her in a big way in this case. It is a pretty big law firm. She is worried because some things they ask her about she cannot remember. She is worried that her bad memory will be held against her. The lawyers are not very nice either and she is intimidated by them. She thinks her own lawyers will sell her out to the corporate lawyers. You know how it works. Please pray for her.

She has so many doctor bills and debts, it's outrageous. She worries constantly about this, and she just prays it will work out in her favor.

I pray your mother is feeling better. Have her use essence of basil for money-drawing purposes. Spiritual-healing baths with *loción de siete machos,* seven male goats' lotion, added to her bath water should help. She should make a small green pouch out of cloth and place *cáscara sagrada,* holy bark, three *ojos de María,* Mary's eyes beans, three *lágrimas de San Pedro,* Saint Peter's tears beans, *semillas de mostaza negra,* black mustard seed, and three *colorines,* red beans, inside the pouch.

She should bless it with Holy Water and carry it with her for money drawing and protection. Finally, pray Psalm 5 for the outcome of court cases. She can find all the items I have requested at any *hierbería.*

Finally, you are going to need spiritual assistance and you should light a candle on your home altar for *Saint Peter of Verona* and to *Saint Ivo* who will send you a powerful lawyer. *Saint Peter's* days are April 6 and 29 while Saint Ivo's day is May 19.

Curanderas are often consulted for court and legal cases that seem insurmountable to the petitioner. As in this case, the woman who has been injured is facing a formidable corporate law firm. Since she is not likely to find adequate help on the physical plane of life, she must enlist support from the spirit world to win.

The *Curandera* recommends that she create a spell for attracting money and for spiritual cleansing. Bathing with spiritual water is an often-prescribed remedy.

Loción siete machos, is a widely-used scented water or florid water used in spiritual healing and rituals. It is one of the most popular spiritual waters. It may be found at any *hierbería.*

The green amulet pouch containing the *cáscara sagrada* herb, sacred husk, three *lágrimas de María* seeds, tears-of-Mary seeds, three *lágrimas de San Pedro, Saint Peter* seeds, black mustard, and three *colorín* seeds are highly recommended for attracting money. *Colorín, lágrimas de María and San Pedro* are seeds found at most *hierberías or botánicas.*

BACK IN COURT
CORRIENDO CORTE

Grandmother, I am requesting your prayer for my entire family. I would also like to request your prayer for my son who is not with me because I have been separated from his mom for a year now. I have not seen my son ever since then and I really do miss him.

I will go to court soon for child support and I really am looking forward to going because I really want my visitation rights as his father to be able to see and be with my son. He is five years old and he needs me.

Please place fresh hen eggs, a head of garlic, lemons and a piedra *alumbre*, alum rock, and leave them on your home altar overnight. The following day, use all those objects to give yourself a *limpia,* or spiritual cleansing, rubbing the egg, or lemon, or garlic head over your body and saying one Our Father and making your petition.

Do this in front of your altar. Pray Psalms 35 and 36. It can be done any day. Dispose of what you use for your cleansing by throwing it outside of your home and yard in the outside garbage can.

Problems of life and family seemingly bury a person who cannot see the proverbial "light at the end of the tunnel." Cultural situations require cultural resolutions. In this case, the *Curandera* recommends fresh hen's eggs, garlic, lemons or piedra alumbre, or alum rock, be placed on an altar overnight.

These are items that are commonly used in cleansing in cases of *susto*, fright sickness, or *mal* de ojo, evil eye, and can be easily located. By placing them on the altar overnight, they pick up or absorb positive spiritual strength. Through these items, the *limpia*, spiritual cleansing ritual, absorbs the bad spirits or negative thoughts from the person's body and transfers them to the objects. The tainted objects must be disposed of outside of the home; preferably at another location.

I'M GOING TO JAIL AGAIN
NUNCA MÁS

Grandmother, thank you for all the work you have done on my mother's behalf. She is home and safe right now. I just pray and have faith that she will come out of this okay. I pray that she never goes back to jail or anywhere even worse.

I have been walking in my faith to the best of my ability. I pray and read my Holy Bible. I believe in the miracles God provides and I have been truly happy. My mother, father, my husband and I, and my two little sisters live in our house together.

One of my sisters is a senior in high school and I just know that she is going to be something wonderful someday. Please pray for her.

We all worry about her. She is never home, is failing school, and feels her friends are the most important thing to her. Please pray for her protection. We really want her to realize how much we love her and how wonderful she is. She is beautiful and smart, she makes friends easily, and she is good to those friends. However, she does not show much respect to my parents, to her teachers or me.

She talks about dropping out of school. We want her to finish high school. She can graduate if she wants to and we know it. She says she hates us and never wants to come home. She says we fight with her all the time. How do we get her to understand and do the things that a young lady should do for her family and her school. We need your help and advice please.

I am attaching a picture of her in case you need it for your prayers. Thank you again for the help you are giving my mother. We love her so much and are so happy she is home.

I also wanted you to know that I have been drug free for months now. I think one of my biggest battles in life was drugs. I really let the drugs get a hold of me. I have turned my life around and, with the power of God; I will stay away from drugs for the rest of my life.

My probation officer gave me a surprise drug screening. It was not instant, though. It was sent off to the lab. That was nearly a month ago and I am scheduled to see her five days from now. Two weeks after that drug screening, I had another screening at my probation office and I passed it and was able to be dismissed from my probation.

I know I have messed up a thousand times in my life, but I have changed. I do not need to go to jail again to learn. This is not like all the other times. I enjoy my life with God. I do not want to do drugs ever again.

I made a promise to never go through that again and I mean it. I know and believe fully that the *Virgen de Guadalupe* has worked a miracle in my life. I know that God and my loved ones have forgiven me of my sins.

Grandmother, now I just battle with the thought of my mistakes coming back to haunt me, and having to go to jail for that first drug screening if it was a bad screening.

Please have mercy on me and pray for me to pass. Please light candles and work magic on my behalf so I can pass. I missed the holidays last year; due to my drug use, I was put in jail. I was there for all the major holidays and missed my baby sister's birthday for the third year in a row. I do not want to put my family through that again.

I truly believe it was a demon that was keeping you on drugs and now that's over. Let me tell you something, you have to be aware of the promises you are making to me.

Please, I always believed in you and I always knew you could do it. Now you have to believe in yourself. You are worthy of being blessed and loved by the spirit of the *Santo Niño de Atocha* who is one of many saints that protect prisoners and help people to stay out of prison. Pray Psalm 71 to keep people out of jail.

You are out of the dark and you will help me pull your sister out of the dark and into the light and happiness of the love of the Holy Spirit of the Lord and Creator. I shall continue to keep your family in my prayers.

Regarding your sister, purchase a packet of dry rosemary and grind it into a powder. Sprinkle a teaspoonful of rosemary powder on the floor on all the corners of your sister's room and one spoonful under the mattress of her bed and leave it there. Call on the Holy Spirit to help you with your petitions for her.

Belief in God and spiritualism are not mutually exclusive with a person's falling into a life which places them at odds with the law. As in this case, the petitioner will most likely spend the rest of her life in and out of jail and abusing drugs.

In between the intermittent episodes when she is out of the judicial system's revolving door, she tries her best to help her family, but always falls back. She is fearful her younger sister is following in her foolhardy footsteps. Grandmother assures her she is genuinely loved by God and blessed by the Holy Spirit in an attempt to keep her on a straight path. The rosemary powder is a spiritual aid intended to protect her sister.

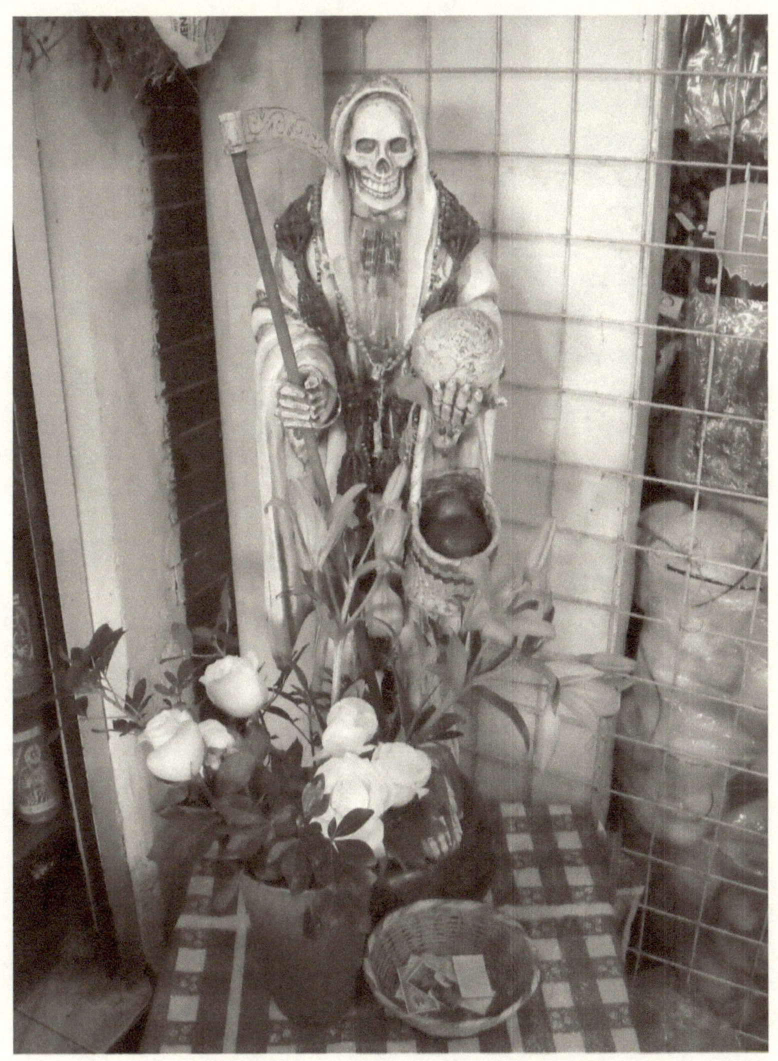

La Santa Muerte is a very Popular Folk Saint

Part 5
The Remedies for the Evil all Around Us

IDENTIFYING SIGNS OF WITCHCRAFT
LAS SEÑALES

How do I know if my problems are caused by a witchcraft spell? To break the spell that has caused you such bad luck due to jealousies, envies and witchcraft that has been cast on you, recite the Prayer of the 12 Truths for nine consecutive days, cleansing your entire body with an alum rock, *piedra alumbre.*

Burn the alum rock after the ninth day and study the rock as it burns, to see if you can see the face of the person who commissioned the witchcraft cast on you formed on the burning alum rock. Pray Psalm 40 to free you of evil spirits and witchcraft.

The *Curandera's* Prayer of the Twelve Truths

To all the stars in the heavens, I ask that you reveal the evil to me. I pray that the spell cast on me will be broken and that I might find the 12 truths that the Lord left for us in this world. I pray that I may be worthy of His love.

- One is the one Holy House in Jerusalem that the Lord left us.
- Two are the two tablets that the Lord gave Moses.
- Three is the Holy Trinity that the Lord gave us.
- Four are the four Gospels that the Lord gave us.
- Five are the five bleeding wounds the Lord suffered as He left the world.
- Six are the six candelabras that are burning on the altar of the Lord.
- Seven are the seven words that the Lord gave us.
- Eight are the eight pleasures that the Lord gave us.
- Nine are the nine months that the Lord was in Mary's womb.

- Ten are the Ten Commandments that the Lord gave us.
- Eleven are the eleven thousand virgins on the altar of the Lord.
- Twelve are the twelve apostles.

May the 13 rays of the sun illuminate my life, along with the 12 apostles; the eleven thousand virgins; the Ten Commandments; the nine months; the eight pleasures; the seven words; the six candelabras; the five wounds; the four Gospels; the Holy Trinity; Moses' two tablets; and the Holy House in Jerusalem.

These are the 12 truths that the Lord left for us in the world. May I be worthy of the precious blood that His body shed for us.

Curanderas believe that maladies originate from both natural and supernatural causes. Illnesses caused by nature may result from a perceived insult to God or a saint. Supernatural illnesses are caused by an agent like witches, *brujas*, or warlocks.

The *Curandera* must first determine if an external agent is involved and this is accomplished by a combination of prayer and by the use of natural remedies.

If the remedy is unsuccessful, it is assumed that the illness or condition has a supernatural origin caused by a person on behalf of a petitioner.

The *Curandera* has provided a prayer that can be used to identify and defeat a problem attributed to witchcraft.

It is not always effective due to some very complicated and tenacious cases, but can be used in conjunction with other remedies with great success.

SMOKING OUT BAD SPIRITS
EL SAHUMERIO

I have noticed that both my home and business have been affected by the negative energies of certain persons who have visited them. Some of these persons, especially in my business, really wish me harm and I fear them and suspect them of doing witchcraft on me.

I remember as a young girl, my grandmother would perform a *sahumerio*, a smoking-house cleansing ritual, on our house after our hateful neighbor came into our home unannounced one time.

I remember that my mother would burn some sort of incense and sprinkle prepared flower water around both our yard and home after our evil neighbor left.

Can you help me prepare and conduct this ritual because both my home and my business need it?

There are many products on the market for the purpose of cleansing and blessing a home or a business with a smoking incense concoction called a *sahumerio*.

Sahumerios are used to rid the home of negative energies, evil influences, unclean spirits and bad emotions.

Sometimes a person might enter a home or business that is clearly unclean, or who leaves behind very negative forces. In cases like this, which are all too common, Holy Water from a church, or sometimes seven churches, is sprinkled around the outside and inside of the home or business.

Successful house blessings require a *sahumerio,* or smoking-ritual cleansing, that could be a single ingredient or multiple ingredients.

For example, a tree or plant resin incense, such as *copal,* mirra, or *estoraque,* or storax, leaf or bark incense as well as other parts of plants such as floral petals are mixed into a *compuesto* with other selected plants for a blending of all the different ingredients.

Specially-selected liquid essences, including *siete machos* and ammonia are also mixed for powerful, aromatic magical blessings that cast out evil influences and attract the assistance of spirits of the light such as angels, saints and folk saints.

My own special blend of *sahumerio,* contains either *copal, estoraque,* or storax, *mirra,* incense along with bay leaves, rosemary, rose petals, ground cinnamon sticks, ground coffee and brown sugar moistened with essence of *narciso negro* or tobacco.

Coffee grounds are also used to bring a lover back. Place three grains of coffee in the palm of your hand in the form of a triangle pointing toward your heart. Recite that your lover will return to you. Say this seven times with your eyes closed. Save the three grains of coffee in a small red bag.

Another popular method of ridding a home or business of bad spirits or to give protection is to place a glass of water with *tomates marinos* in the home or business. These seeds are both male and female, and you must have one of each in the water.

I have found this to be a very powerful and effective cleansing, and blessing method with spiritual medicine.

Always pray while applying the ritual to the house or business.

Spiritual cleansings of businesses or homes and their continuous protection are the most frequent rituals performed by *Curanderas*.

One of the most impressive experiences I have ever had was a request to bring a *Curandera* to the home of a very infamous witch, or *bruja*, who had recently died.

Her family was afraid to venture into her home until it had been cleansed of all its evil spirits. Not knowing what to expect, I don't think I have ever been so scared.

In fact, the *Curandera* had a very difficult time with the cleansing because it lasted four or five hours. She cleaned each nook and cranny of the tainted house, and when we finally left, we could feel the difference. The house had been cleansed of all evil spirits.

Grandmother always recommends special smudging the home to repel evil spells and to purify and attract good.

The following are herbal smudges, a special contribution on herbal smudging from Reynaldo Lopez a member of the Mision Fidencista Batallón de David:

Smudge orange peel to attract happiness

Smudge tomatillo to attract money

Smudge cilantro to attract loyalty

Smudge salvia to purify and renew energy

Smudge sunflower seeds and sugar to attract abundancia

Smudge artemisa to have clairvoyance and lucid dreams

Smudge coffee grounds to scare bad spirits

Smudge rosemary to eliminate illness caused by viruses

Smudge lavender to bring calm and tranquility

Smudge chamomile to eliminate spells and bring luck

Smudge mint to calm the nerves

Smudge laurel to end nerves and protect from spells

Smudge cinnamon sticks to improve a relationship and attract abundance

Smudge aromatic cloves in order to eliminate gossip and attract good luck, money and good friends and expel bad spirits

Smudge garlic to rid envy and do it on Fridays to attract money

Smudge white rose to bring about harmony and love

Smudge tabaco to eliminate evil spiritist

Smudge palo santo to purify and protect

Smudge star anis to protect from the evil eye and bring protection and good luck

Smudge rue to end bad vibes

Smudge manderina husk to attract a new romance

Smudge bark of the oak to attract fertility

Smudge limon grass to energize talismans

Smudge eucalyptus leaves to repel bad people

Smudge guinea hen weed to attract a job and make your dreams come true

Smudge violet petals to cure a broken heart

KNOWING BAD OMENS
LECHUZA Y BUEN AGÜEROS

Grandmother, Last night I had a vision and I could see all the candles I had lit for the Holy Spirit over the years. It was a magical experience. Then suddenly I noticed a bird flying in my darkened kitchen and it landed at the foot of my bed. I noticed that it was a white dove. I tried and tried to drive it out of my house, but as I opened the back door a hummingbird flew into my kitchen.

I awoke to the sound of my son coughing. What does it mean? Does this have a spiritual meaning or special message for me?

First, I need total clarity from you. Did you have a vision that is a supernatural sight while awake, or did you have a dream while asleep?

Angels often take the form of birds both good and evil. When they manifest to humankind, while awake or in their sleep, they are often seen as birds. Both doves and hummingbirds are considered good. The good ones are the Creator's messengers.

I believe that you are receiving a message, so you need to try to understand it. If it is a spiritual message, it will continue and the message will proceed through its own symbolism. Be sure to have a notepad next to your bed and write everything down that you dream.

Only you can understand the Creator's messages, so be ready for them. I believe you should carry out ritual cleansings, or *limpias,* seven Fridays in a row and pray Psalm 23 to keep you safe from evil.

It is normal for people to dream a cornucopia of spiritual images. Dreams are not always spiritual messages, but often they are.

The *Curandera* informs the petitioner that doves and hummingbirds are considered good omens, or *buen agüeros,* but there are also *agüeros malos*, or bad omens.

Omen acceptance is part of every culture and, often, the person who believes that they have witnessed an omen will ask the *Curandera* for an interpretation.

Most dreams, however, must be interpreted in sequence over time. A record of dreams is always a good idea and it assists the *Curandera*, the dreamer and or counselor with an accurate interpretation.

Owls, or *lechuzas*, are common symbolic and, but often do. *Curanderismo* believes that shapeshifting entities in *Curanderismo*. They do not always convey negativity evil witches can "shape shift," changing their form into that of an owl or other birds and animals.

It's always advisable to cleanse oneself and each family member to rid the body and the home of negative influences.

In this case, just to be sure, the *Curandera* recommends repeating *limpias*, or ritual cleansings, for seven Fridays in a row.

SCARED OF THE UNSEEN
EL MIEDOSO

Grandmother, I am writing to you about a child. He seems to get scared very easily even though no one tries to frighten him. He sees things in the house that we cannot see that scare him. He gets so scared that he holds or loses his breath and he pees every time this happens to him, and it happens often.

In the beginning, he would get scared with any little noise, and now it can happen without any noise at all. When there is no one present, he jumps up and kick, and then punches the air like if he is trying to fight off something or someone unseen. He is definitely seeing something we can't see.

Can you tell me what he sees? What is scaring him? What is he trying to fight off? Like I said before, after this occurs, he seems to lose his breath and looks like he cannot breathe. Can you please let me know what is scaring my nephew or more importantly, how can we help or protect him? Should we have our home and his room cleansed?

Is he an only child? How long has he been so easily scared? Do you think he has panic attacks or seizures? Have you tried treating him for fright sickness, or *susto,* or for some other trauma? Is he on any kind of medication? What is his age? Has he been checked by a physician?

It is important that I know these things. Is he allergic to anything? Please let me know as much as possible, so that I may be able to try to determine what's bothering him. Then I will see if there is something we might be able to do for his treatment and well-being from his symptoms. Pray Psalm 10 to overcome all evil spirits.

Children are often believed to be able to see and hear things that as adults we cannot. This may be true, especially if the child is visibly fearful of things unseen.

The *Curandera* asks about any physical ailments. If no malady exists, then the *Curandera* would prescribe that the child receives a ritual cleansing, or limpia, and that the home be cleansed spiritually as well, with a *despojo* or spiritual cleansing.

TOAD SPELL
EL SAPO TONTO

Grandmother, I am wondering if you can help me. A young woman has put a spell on my husband. She has a spell on him that makes him treat me very badly, and he refuses anyone but her. I know you may wonder how I know this, and I am not sure what to tell you. I just do.

The spell has gotten to the point where I just got fed up and walked out of the room to get away from him. I believe that is exactly what she wants me to do so that he will have a reason to leave me or have me leave him. Either way, the situation is desperate. We had a very good marriage before this woman showed up.

Please light a seven-day votive candle to *San Alejo* and another to *San Ignacio de Loyola* with your husband's photo under a clear glass of water between both candles to cleanse him of the spell that she has placed over him. Remember that at most *hierberías* there are preprepared candles and other products, like sprays, that can be used in the home against witchcraft.

It is prevalent in *Hispanic* culture for spells to be used in fixing and breaking relationships. In many cases, if not most, they are harmless, but some are very evil.

The *Curandera* recommends a primary-level reversing spell to determine if any evil is intended. Some spells, or *trabajos*, performed by competent witches and *brujas,* may attempt serious harm or death to the party on which the spell has been cast.

In fact, there are documented cases of spiritual, warfare taking place between witches and *Curanderas* that proceed for years without end or until one of them dies. In this case, the *Curandera* recommended a first-level reversing spell to discover any evil intentions.

Once witchcraft spells have been created as "works," or *trabajos,* they are placed somewhere for safekeeping depending upon the requirement of the spell.

Often, they are hidden or secretly buried in an intended victim's yard or business. Sometimes they are disposed of in water, like a river, or are thrown into the sea. Extremely evil works of witchcraft which are intended to take someone's life are often placed in cemeteries.

It is not uncommon for the witch, or *bruja,* to seal away the witchcraft job and sometimes items care placed in the mouth of a live toad and the toad's mouth is sewn shut. This action represents sure death for the innocent toad and the completion of the evil intent of the witchcraft spell.

THE HECHICERA
EL CLARIVIDENTE

Grandmother, please help me in my situation with my boyfriend, if you could. I told you that he left me. Well, I have been talking to this person who can read people's minds. So far, everything she has told me has come true. She claims that she is not a witch and that she only uses her powers to help people. But it scares me a little because if she can cast good spells, she can certainly cast bad ones as well.

This mind reader told me that my boyfriend left me because he has a lot of stress in his life and that I give him more stress. He claims that I am a control freak.

The mind reader told me that if we could take away all of his other stresses and leave only the one that I cause him, that it would not be enough to drive him away from me. But it sounds very strangely like witchcraft.

I don't want him in my life if I have to resort to witchcraft to get him. It is just so easy for him to blame all of his stress on me, rather than, for him to accept that all of these other problems are causing his stress, which I have nothing to do with. I just wanted to know if there is a way to help him clear his mind because I am afraid that he could have a nervous breakdown.

I shall try to do what I can for you. Why do you really think your boyfriend left you? What does this psychic spiritual advisor tell you is going to happen?

Will she be able to help you with your dilemma and if yes, why are you contacting me? Did she ask you to change your behavior in order to get him to come back to you? Would he be willing to seek help?

Please bring me a recent picture of him and of yourself, if you are willing for me to help you, so that I may keep both of you in my prayers. You may light a *San Alejo* and a *San Ignacio de Loyola* candle for their spirits to come to him and for you to cleanse yourself of confusion, evil and negative energies. Also, have either of you considered seeing a counselor?

In the *Hispanic* community there are many people who claim to be able to cast spells to reunite lovers. It is never advisable to undertake this even though it may be very tempting.

Many people you encounter will tell you that they have done it and that it has worked. This activity falls into the context of witchcraft; believed to be revisited upon the petitioner.

However, there is always a price to pay for delving into magic. You don't know nor understand the forces that are being utilized to bring about the desired effect and the heavy price you may pay. The returning sweetheart may exhibit negative personality changes as a result of the interference with his or her free will by the manipulating spirits.

DARK SHADOWS
UNA SOMBRA NEGRA

Grandmother, my mom saw you recently. She informed me that she had given you pictures of me and my boyfriend and that I could contact you if I needed to.

I am asking if you can help me out with a situation that has been taking place in my apartment. Ever since I moved in here, strange things have been taking place. I have trouble sleeping and I wake up every night around the same time, only to feel as though someone is staring at me from the doorway of my bedroom.

On one occasion, I woke up as usual and saw a shadowy, childlike figure in the doorway. Then, a few nights later, my boyfriend was sitting on the bed and he felt a hand pressing down on his head but there was no one around. We were the only ones in the apartment.

We have also had very strange dreams. I dreamt that I was possessed by something evil. He has also had similar but more disturbing dreams. He had a dream that there was a little boy standing in the center of our bedroom and that he was trying to harm me. My boyfriend wanted to stop the little boy but could not grab anything. It was a ghost.

My boyfriend dreamt that his brother was in our apartment but it really was not him, it was something pretending to be his brother.

About two weeks ago, my boyfriend woke up in the middle of the night and saw a dark shadow-figure standing over me with its arms raised. When he tried to reach for it, it disappeared. Last night he dreamt that his evil twin, was pacing back and forth in front of our bedroom door staring back at him.

I would like to know if there is anything I could do to make all of this go away. I have tried Holy Water, but it only helps for about three weeks; then things start to happen again. If there is any advice as to what is causing this or how I can make this go away, please let me know. Any advice you can give us will be very much appreciated.

To cleanse the apartment and yourselves of ghosts or evil spirits or entities, burn incense, myrrh, and *copal* incense in the apartment to cleanse it and your physical persons as well.

Getting rid of evil is often difficult, so enlist the help of *San Mauricio, San Cipriano* and *San Cristóbal,* all three are used to rid evil spirits. You must also perform repeated spiritual cleansings and pray Psalm 17 to stay safe from evil.

Many persons believe that spirits, including evil ones, can be invited into the home inadvertently. The spirits might enter attached to an object that one might acquire, at a second-hand store. Additionally, spirits will attach themselves to a person and be brought into the home.

Sometimes the spirit, may be harmless, it simply resides in the home and existed there years before you arrived. In any case, the home and the people who live there must be cleansed and only a competent *Curandera* may adequately perform this ritual.

CHARMED
TRABAJÁNDOME

Today, a woman came to my place of employment. She stopped at the guard shack and told them that I had told her to come and sell *burritos,* so they let her through and told her what building I was in.

When she walked in, she asked someone to point me out to her. She did not know me and I do not know her. I certainly did not tell her to come and sell *burritos*. She did not know who I was and I felt sorry for her so I bought some of her *burritos* and ate them.

I now know that I was very stupid to do that. I am sure now that I ate some kind of witchcraft. The more I think about it, the more terrorized I become.

I'm very scared because I realized that someone is trying to hurt me by witchcraft. It is a very strange feeling. I am now imagining that something is growing inside me.

She made it seem to the people at the guard shack that she knew me when she did not. It is obvious that someone sent her. Was she the messenger of death? Am I just being paranoid or is something very bad happening? Please help me or am I just freaking out over nothing?

This sounds very mysterious and horrible! Who do you think would do this to you? Maybe it was just her tactic to be allowed permission to enter certain gated work sites. Otherwise, she might never be allowed in. It is very probable that she knew exactly who you were, even though she pretended not to know you.

In situations like this most often the messenger has been given your photo. You didn't meet the actual witch. You probably met a demon messenger. Are you positive you do not know who she is? It is very strange.

I do understand why you would feel sorry for her, which is part of the spell they placed on you so you would eat what they gave you.

Do you understand why someone might be trying to do witchcraft on you? Someone gave her your name with instructions to sell you some *burritos* with poison or witchcraft powder in them.

Then on the other hand, it could be nothing. It sounds like you need to be very careful not to ever eat food from someone you don't know. Someone may be trying to hurt you and it simply is not sanitary. It is very important that you let me know immediately if anything else happens.

Say a special prayer to *San Cipriano* to assist you and pray Psalm 145 to keep ghosts and spirits away from you.

This is troublesome. It's quite evident someone visited the petitioner's workplace, lied to gain entry, and convinced the person to eat something of unknown origin.

Hispanic culture in general, always tells its people never accept food from someone you do not know for fear that something has been placed in it with evil intent.

The *Curandera* offers good advice. When in doubt about food: always politely decline. If a person is hungry, it may be difficult to refuse but not if it's food you purchase. Caution and vigilance are always the best preventative measures.

WITCHCRAFT DOLLS
MUÑECOS

When I go to my local *hierbería*, I see a whole section with very ugly witchcraft dolls, *munecas*. Some are made of cloth and others are made of wax. Some are genderless rag dolls and others are very anatomically correct female and male wax candle dolls.

Whenever I ask the woman there about these dolls and what they are for, she instantly changes the subject. The most I have been able to get out of her is "if you don't know what they are for, then you don't need them."

I have gone to several mail-order websites which sell them in all types, sizes, materials and colors. I simply want an explanation of what they are for and how they are used.

The *hierbería* or *botánica* is first and foremost a business. Therefore, they need sales. Sales are determined by the market and they stock the things that people ask for most. So *hierberías* and *botánicas* stock items for many different spiritual purposes, beliefs and traditions. The items stocked in these stores are for both *Curanderismo* for *santería* and witchcraft, and the dolls and fetishes are for spell casting or hexing.

Both the cloth dolls, wax dolls or candles in human form are used in witchcraft and hexing rituals. They are not evil by themselves but when they are "worked," or spiritually activated they can be very dangerous.

Never touch one that you see or encounter with your bare hands. Pray Psalms 67 and 68 to keep evil from imprisoning you in a doll.

Seeing a witchcraft doll in a store for the first time can be shocking, but what is more disconcerting is the discovery of these items after they have been prepared and used in a witchcraft spell intended to do someone harm or placed in your home or yard.

When they are completed, they may contain human hair and substances as well as personal clothing. As shown in the National Geographic documentary series "Taboo: Mexican Witchcraft," *Hispanic* witchcraft can and does seek to destroy marriages, and even kill.

Not knowing what forces are used to bring forth the spell, these items of Mexican witchcraft should always be considered very dangerous.

BEDEVILED
MALDICIÓN

I believe I was cursed as an infant because my grandmother was a *Curandera* and had many enemies. When I was about three years old, I woke in the middle of the night and saw a fireball over my bed. I remember it well. The next day, our house burned to the ground. I have had a lot of bad luck in every aspect of my life, personal, business and health.

Doctors have told me repeatedly that there is nothing wrong with me, but I still have this feeling that I have inherited a curse.

Please help me. I do not want to cry anymore or live in fear. I want to live a healthy, normal life and I would like to have some good luck for a change.

It is likely that you are a continued recipient of your grandmother's curse, that is your grandmother's curse has been passed on to you. I have seen this many times where curses are passed on to children and grandchildren.

If your grandmother was cursed by her enemies, as you say, the curse falls on the rest of the family for generations to come. You must find a way to end the curse.

The fireball you witnessed was a spirit messenger, either sent to warn you or to protect you from what was about to happen. You were, and probably still are, being watched over and protected by some entity; maybe the spirit of your grandmother.

I believe you were born with a special mission in life, to serve others in some divine capacity. That is why you were not in the house when it burned down.

I would say that your survival is an example of Divine Providence and evidence that you are indeed protected. But Divine Providence is not good luck. They are very different things. I believe the doctors are correct, this is not a physical ailment. It is a spiritual issue.

I don't think that there is anything physically or psychologically wrong with you. You will have to protect yourself for the rest of your life from this curse, unless you can find someone powerful enough to break it.

A family curse is a common concept within the *Hispanic* cultural and familial fabric. This is especially true in families with an ancestor or family member who practices or used to practice *Curanderismo* or *brujería*. *Curanderismo*, as other cultural dogmas, definitely acknowledges that curses can be passed down from generation to generation.

THE SORCERER
LA BRUJA

Grandmother, the reason I asked for your help is because I hoped you would help remove this woman from my ex-husband's home and, with God's help, he will come back home to me.

As I explained, there is this woman who has paid someone a lot of money so she can remain in my ex-husband's house. She is still paying someone to help her. As long as she is in the picture and doing these bad things, the situation between me and my husband will not improve. One day he is fine, and the next day he is different and will not even talk to me.

I need to remove this woman and all the witchcraft from my life. With God's help and the Holy Spirit, I have faith that things will improve.

I am sorry if I did not fully explain myself about what I wanted. I just want this woman to go away. I know in my heart that if she is gone, he will come home to me.

This is the first time in all the years we have been together that this has ever happened. All I want to know is if you see any hope that things will get better, and if you can remove this woman from his house.

First, you must cleanse yourself with spiritual-blessing baths. Boil rice and use the water in your bath water for at least three Fridays in a row. Use the same boiled rice to sprinkle outside around your house, calling on the celestial spirits of light to favor you and approve your petition.

After that, you must burn a red wax candle with a glass of water over his picture at your bedside. You will call out his name three times near the glass of water in a longing fashion. Do this at 3 a.m. for as many early mornings as the candle is lit.

Soon after you do this, he will come to you. When he does, you will give him the same glass of water to drink out of. This will deliver him from all of her spells.

Finally, light a Saint Michael Archangel candle and implore the archangel to assist you to vanquish the other woman from this spiritual war you are in.

If you are able to acquire any object of hers, burn it and then bury it in a jar in your yard. Once she is enclosed, she will never bother you again.

Beware! Realize that the most common type of witchcraft is to experience a curse placed on a former spouse or lover.

Many practicing *brujas* or witches are consumed by this business; casting no other spells, only those affecting relationships. Due to this ongoing witchcraft, it is always wise to be protected with a special amulet or talisman prepared by a magic ritual.

Always be sure to cleanse yourself and your home; protecting the family unit and marriage in order to avoid problematic situations.

FEAR DARKNESS
LAS TINIEBLAS

Regarding my nephew, things are a little better but the situation is very stressful on my sister. Now, the doctors say she has arthritis in her neck from the whiplash she got when she was in a car accident last year.

She's not doing well, and I also think someone did something very evil to her because she told me that she has seen a black shadow at the back door, and continues to see a *lechuza,* or owl, when dropping her son off at work.

My sister has been afraid to talk about her experiences, but now tells us that this black shadow person comes to have sex with her and she says that it's an ongoing experience. Please help me because I think someone is trying to drive her crazy. She is not herself and we need your help.

I don't understand why you think someone would be trying to drive her crazy. All three of you should take a head of garlic and rub it all over your body, cleansing it of negative and evil forces and energies that bring about suffering and bad happenings to your sister.

Say an Our Father when performing these cleansing rituals and say a special prayer to *San Cristóbal*, the patron saint against evil spirits. But most importantly, you need to settle down and find rational explanations for the things that you say are happening to her. Your sister must place a Holy relic above the head of her bed to ward off he errant incubus, or male devil she says is having sex with her.

Throw the head of garlic in the trash when you are done with the *limpias*. Repeat the *limpias* for seven consecutive Fridays. Start with one today, even though it is not Friday, for urgency reasons. Sprinkle rice and wheat seed with Holy Water around the house for protection and for prosperity.

Do this the first day of each month. On the last day of each month, burn special *copal* incense in your home to further cleanse it. You should also consider a complete *sahumerio* or smoking *limpia*, of your home. This will cleanse the house of evil curses and negative energies that may have entered the home and especially the shadow man if he truly exists.

Hispanics frequently have latent recollections of events and experiences, especially if they are of a spiritual or supernatural nature. In this case, it was verified that the petitioner has suppressed memories of sexual abuse as a child.

From the testimony it seems that this woman has fully comprehended *Curanderismo* and witchcraft most of her life. The appearance of a spirit (incubus or succubus) who has sex with someone is not uncommon in the life of a person encompassed by the supernatural.

One aspect of the spirit world attracts others. The attraction, the sexual abuse, the repressed memories are not always benign. Especially in this case, it seems that the sister needs ongoing treatment and support.

EXORCISING DEMONS
SACANDO DEMONIOS

Grandmother, I am a Catholic, and recently our parish priest talked about persons possessed by demons and he says that the church has special rituals to cast them out.

I was talking to my friend about this, who is a Protestant, and she says that her church also performs exorcisms from time to time when her pastor believes that someone is demon possessed.

Can a *Curandera* cast out demons also? I have heard that they can. Finally, how do you know when a person is demon possessed, are there any tests or signs?

Early in my experience a woman brought her niece for me to examine. Her niece had been ill and was under a doctor's care. The doctor had examined her and had run every kind of test, finding nothing wrong her. The young adolescent girl continued to be ill for seven months before she was brought to me.

On the surface, she seemed to be okay to me, but other than that, she was a little reluctant to see me or allow me to place my hands on her. She appeared to be uncomfortable or uneasy around me.

I immediately sensed that there was something evil deep inside her. I could see it looking back at me when I looked deep into her eyes.

I blessed a Holy Rosary and a *Cruz de Caravaca* for her to wear around her neck. These blessed items would protect her against evil spirits.

I also asked that her aunt see to it that her niece drink a cup of tea daily made from three herbs: *peonía, tumba vaquero* and *perejil*. The concoction is intended to provoke the expulsion of the fluids that form in the stomach lining from the manifestation of any unclean spirit living in her body and making her ill.

After my examination, her aunt drove the niece home, but before they arrived, the niece flew into an uncontrollable rage. In a terrible fit in the car, she tore the Rosary and *Cruz de Caravaca* from around her neck and threw them out the window.

Once home, her mother and aunts prepared the tea I recommended, and gave her a cup to drink. I was then called and asked if I was able to go to their home to perform a cleansing and healing ritual. Since I lived nearby, I was able to go and I arrived just a few minutes later.

Entering the home, I gasped at what I saw. Several of her relatives were holding the girl down on the floor. It was then that I fully encountered what I had suspected from her initial visit. The young woman was demonically possessed and by a formidable demon.

I asked the family if they had contacted their family priest or minister. They indicated that a local priest had come by their home earlier in the week, but not prepared for what he found or trained as an exorcist, he quickly fled their house scared to death.

They said that he would never come back. Knowing the priest personally, I called him and informed him of the situation with his parishioner. I told him I was going to pray for the girl and asked him for his blessing, for his prayers, and for my protection, and for that of the family.

I performed the exorcism rituals on the girl as I have learned to do, and during this process I learned that she had started acting strangely after a visit to the cemetery with her aunts to pray at her grandfather's grave on Father's Day. That was seven months ago.

I was told that at the moment when she passed through the cemetery's gate, she accidentally stepped on a witchcraft object that had been placed on the ground.

After that, I was told that she appeared to be in a daze, in some altered state and became incoherent. During the exorcism sessions, I also learned that seven months before this event occurred, her parents were awakened in the middle of the night by their daughter's screams. She told them that two demons had come into her bedroom through a window and had sex with her.

I worked with this young girl, day in and day out, for more than four months. Finally, I was able to cast out a number of demonic spirits, asking each of them to identify themselves by name.

Some of those, especially a very powerful and evil spirit, would keep returning to the girl's body refusing to leave permanently.

This happened several times until it could no longer overcome the exorcism. The exorcism was eventually successful and the young girl was relieved from her torment, confusion, unrest and illness. A year later, she seemed to be fine and had no further incidences with evil spirits.

Exorcising demons is an officially sanctioned rite of the Catholic Church. In Catholicism it is only performed by a person who is trained and approved by the bishop of a diocese. Exorcism is also a routine function of evangelical religions and their ministers, and a known practice of *Curanderas.*

Another method which followers of *Curanderismo* use to shun and cast out devils is to call upon the assistance of *San Cipriano, San Alejo or San Ignacio.*

They light a candle to *San Miguel Arcángel* and place it inside a vessel containing an inch of dirt along with an inch of Holy Water.

After a person takes their loved one to see a *Curandera* for an exorcism that act should always be followed up by a trip to seek professional help as well. Very likely, the person will require ongoing assistance from both *Curandera* and medical professional.

TORMENTED
ATORMENTADO

Grandmother, can you help me to understand the healing baths? I have been suffering for a long time and have been tormented by the devil all of my life. I can sense that my life is going to end soon.

God has called me to do great things with my life, and healing me from this awful disease that has been cast upon me is one of the first things I'm going to accomplish with your help.

Try boiling rue, rosemary and basil, and bathe with the water on Mondays and Fridays at high noon. Do this for seven straight weeks praying and making your petition to the Lord God.

It will be a stronger healing if you are able to find and burn the *San Alejo* and the *San Ignacio de Loyola* candles for 40 straight days. You must place your photograph between both candles and a clear glass of water over your photo.

I pray you can be patient with me so that I may try to help you. If you are unable to be patient with me, I will understand and I will respect you for that and will step aside if you want me to.

All I can do for anyone is try my best. If that is not good enough, then let that be the will of God. I, for one, will have to accept that.

First of all, the *Curandera* did not answer your question of "what are the baths for?" The *Curandera* senses something else is at work here or the petitioner has a hidden agenda.

While this may have been answered in another correspondence between the two, the petitioner is a suffering hypochondriac, and therefore, experiences imaginary maladies and suspects every remedy. Therefore, the petitioner will not rest until the question on the baths is answered. Simply stated, spiritual baths wash away negative energies.

Be wary of persons who have spent their lives living with hypochondria and who jump from one religion or from healer to healer. They can never be satisfied and never find relief because of their mental illness.

Because their lives are surrounded by their so-called physical ailments, they never want to hear the truth that it is all in their minds. Any healer, therapist, reader and/ or counselor can become exhausted or ill when a demanding hypochondriac visits too frequently.

The hypochondriacs will wear the healer out; then disappear when they feel that they have milked the healer for everything she has. Then they just move on to another healer and are never heard from again. At some point, it becomes necessary to end the sessions to preserve the healer's own emotional and physical health.

WHITE WITCHCRAFT
LA HECHICERA

Grandmother, thank you for your suggested remedy for my previous request. I really like the remedy that uses the different waters and the goat's milk. I have a friend who can get me the sea and river water, but I will have to wait a few months for it to arrive.

A woman put a *brujería* hex on my aunt that will not allow her to ever go back to her home. If she steps a foot inside her hometown, she will surely die.

My aunt told me that a woman buried her hair and clothes in cemetery dirt and other evil stuff in a jar and buried it in my aunt's hometown. That ritual act captures her spirit in that place until it is released.

My aunt is a famous *bruja*, witch in the town, and she has been at war with other witches all her life. They are in a standoff right now, but have successfully prevented my aunt from going home.

To make matters worse, I believe my aunt has used my photo and hair as well as my clothes to do witchcraft on me. She is upset that I don't want to be trained as a *bruja* before she dies. It is even more evil than that. She wants me to carry on the war with the other *brujas,* witches, and I don't want that kind of life. So now, my aunt has turned against me. I need help in defeating her because she is a very powerful and famous *bruja*.

Stay away from your aunt until you are able to resolve this issue with her. Yes, there are many possible ways of breaking witchcraft. I will prepare a very special and most powerful prayer to have witchcraft removed from you. Trust in the Holy Spirit.

To undo the witchcraft that has been done to you, you must take seven baths on seven consecutive Fridays.

On the first Friday, bathe with water from a river. If you are able add the leaves of the Alamo tree to your bath. The Alamo removes all negative influences from the body. The second Friday, bathe with water from underground, like water from a spring or a well. The third Friday, bathe in rainwater. The fourth Friday, bathe in lake water. The fifth Friday, bathe with Holy Water, that must be from a Catholic Church. The sixth Friday, bathe with seven liters of goat's milk. The seventh Friday, bathe with three gallons of water from the sea. With each spiritual bath, you will receive a healing and by the seventh bath, the spell will be broken.

After seven weeks, your aunt's witchcraft will no longer make you suffer and you will have defeated her. As a witch, she will know this and have more respect for you, but she is going to want to know my name and you should divulge that.

In the United States and in Mexico, I have met persons who claim to have grandmothers and grandfathers who were either healers and *Curanderas* or witches *brujas*.

While this may be true, the descendant and their tales can become self-fulfilling prophecies in the lives of their descendants. The younger generation lives in the shadow of its ancestor and believes that it must carry on this war of the witches. This is simply not true. This leads to the absorbing of all sorts of spiritual and supernatural burdens, imagined health issues, and convoluted magical problems.

SPELL BOUND
EMBRUJADA

Thank you for your kindness. I truly appreciate you and I will be patient. I'm just so used to people forgetting about or not caring at all about me. I'm so relieved I have your help and I'm thankful for your understanding. I'm at a difficult time in my life right now. I am trying my hardest to receive what the Lord has in store for me so I can begin my new life in the spirit.

I feel that this agonizing back and neck problem I have is the only way the devil has power over me. I'm growing spiritually and just surrendered my life to the Lord this year. I'm not giving up on my healing so the devil can have his way.

My faith has grown so much and I have come a long way before I got in contact with you. I'm just tired of all the evil in the world and in my family.

I care very much about your spirituality and have great respect for you. If you have placed your life in the Lord's hands, the devil may tempt you, but he cannot touch you if you don't let him.

Evil will not go away. It must be defeated. It is one's own responsibility to have the faith, strength and valor to combat evil. You need to allow God to help you through those around you, and pray that God may bless those who hurt you. Pray that He allow those who can help you to be near you and set apart from you those who want to hurt you.

Find a special prayer to reverse the spell against you or a *rompe trabajo*, break a spell. You will know when you have found the prayer for you. Give yourself cleansing baths with healing herbs such as rosemary, anise seed and star anise, basil and myrrh.

Be sure to have a High John the Conqueror oil, spray or candle in your home and use it frequently by spraying it in the rooms that you are in the most such as your bedroom.

People sometimes blame God for their bad luck or life's conditions. While bad luck will continue to be the most common blame, the truth is that people must think seriously about becoming spiritual while developing faith. Try not to allow evil to enter your thoughts and always remember that "an idle mind is the devil's workshop."

Some people believe that they inherently have bad luck or are *salados,* or salted. They are so convinced that they have bad luck, that they obsess over it, and that causes them to make bad decisions and worsens their situation.

If one feels this way, one should wear an amulet or talisman to prevent it. Then, purchase candles and other objects in the hierberías to reverse bad luck. Sometimes they are easily taken advantage of by commercial *Curanderas.*

ANCESTORAL CURSE
ESPANTADO

Grandmother, these last two days I have been very confused about God and I am very nervous. I have been seeking help from a man who practices *Santería.*

I feel that I am constantly being attacked by evil spirits and my schizophrenia has returned. This Brazilian man told me that I am a spirit medium and that is why I am suffering spirit attacks. He says that if I turn my back on my calling, I will go crazy, become *trastornado.* Please send some much-needed advice. I feel that I am also under attack by witches.

On the one hand, I am told that I am being called to become a *Curandera,* while on the other; witches are trying to keep me from my spiritual development, or *desarrollo espiritual.* I do not even know what that is.

Seeking spiritual help from a variety of religious belief systems can lead to confusion and I think that is where you are. Keep the faith in a higher power, a supreme being you can always count on to be there for you in your hour of need. Place your life in God's hands and go on about living your life as best as you can. The sacred faith you place in Him will see you through your journey. You will be fine. I am your friend in prayer.

There are many different religions and sects which surround us. Most offer support for humanity's multitudinous problems. In this case, the petitioner has encountered a practitioner of *Afro-Brazilian* or *Afro-Caribbean* practices.

Since these practices are based on spirit possession and trance-induced states, any cult that relies on spirit possession may be misdiagnosed as schizophrenic.

This petitioner claims to have schizophrenia and, therefore, is easy prey for cults.

The *santero* probably thinks that the person is a trance medium in training but in fact has a mental condition. Since many of these practices are based upon trance-induced states, spirit possession, as well as drugged stupors, they resemble cults and not religions.

Obviously, exceptions exist. Any group that insists that all members commit an act that causes fear, confusion and shame is highly destructive. Losing one's sense of self and connection to right and wrong is the first warning sign.

THE CONJURE
EL CONJURO

Grandmother, some of my friends and family members have put evil spells on me for about 30 years now and nothing I can do will take them off. Right now, I am suffering from extreme jealousy, envy and hatred from anyone that sets eyes on me. It is a very complex spell. To break or romper envy, use the *Piedra Alumbre* along with lemon drops and *Siete Machos loción*.

I have a very long list of people who hate me and want to do me harm. Please pray a special prayer for me. Please help me break these evil spells that have ruined my life.

You may start healing and reversing the evil spells by putting one tablespoon of salt and one ounce of rubbing alcohol in a pail of rain water, and bathe with that for nine straight Fridays. While you do this, complete your prayer to *San Cipriano*. You must pray to the healing spirits of light for blessings. Never give up. This might also be a spiritual test to see if you are worthy. Fight back against evil.

Envy and jealousy amongst friends and family members is very common. It is not unusual for family members to place or to arrange spells to be placed upon other family members and to carry on lengthy vendettas or to seek revenge, *venganza*.

The fact that this person feels that everyone hates him is a sign of deep-seated problems and he believes he has been falsely judged, or *perjuicio*.

Often, the failure to receive therapy results in the continued reaction or feeling that everyone is against them. Research has shown that counseling over time with a *Curandera* can be a very effective treatment for an ongoing mental or emotional issue.

EVIL IS ALL AROUND
PERSEGUIDO

Grandmother, I feel that there are those that wish for me to fail in everything I do. I am about to begin working as a pre-kindergarten teacher, but I have already started off on the wrong foot. I believe that it is because people envy my success and the education that I have attained against all odds. I am the only person in my family that is educated.

I have been cursed with bad luck with money and especially with love. I am a great believer that there are those who have the spiritual *don*, or gift. I know that the spirits can do both good and bad. Is there something that I can do to protect myself from envy and evil?

Cleanse yourself by doing a *limpia,* ritual cleansing, with a handful of *gobernadora,* creosote bush, or a bunch of fresh parsley, rubbing it over your entire body saying a prayer and making your petition to your spirit guide and protector, or guardian angel. Do this on the last day of each month.

Many *Hispanics* feel that they must consult a *Curandera* if they suffer from loneliness and believe that the whole world is against them.

All aspects of so-called bad luck are interpreted as evil spirits or spells cast against them when it is not necessarily the case. Sometimes life and challenges are our own soul's desire to grow strong. Cultural foundations are much stronger than educational achievements and one's personal level of educational achievement does not eliminate the need to enlist spiritual aid through a *Curandera.*

PINS AND NEEDLES
ALFILERES

Grandmother, I'm writing to let you know how things are going. We have been performing the egg cleansing ritual that you prescribed. Today is the third day in a row that we have performed the hex-breaking ritual with the egg on our poor innocent child. Each time we break the fresh egg after the *limpia,* or spiritual cleansing, the contents of the egg is rotten and full of little things that look like straight pins. It's ugly and horrible and it stinks.

The truth is that we are very scared because we don't have any enemies that we know of. We don't have many friends either.

We are homebodies and live in a small town. There are some people here that have animals such as cows and chickens, so I didn't have any trouble getting the fresh eggs.

I don't know who would hate us so much that they would want to cause extreme harm to a child. I understand that it could be coming from someone in our former town and the evil has followed us.

One day I walked out of my house and noticed an egg had been thrown at my car. On another occasion, on the front door of my house, there was some kind of powder or *polvo* that looked like ashes.

It seems that someone here is trying to scare us or really has done something very awful to our child. I don't understand why, unless they have been sent from someplace else.

Get nine fresh farm eggs from someone you can trust. The ones they sell at the stores are not fresh. These have to come right from under the hen and in the morning if at all possible.

Recite the Lord's Prayer as you pass the egg along the child's body in a sweeping motion early in the morning. The child could even be asleep. Be sure that you hold the egg in your right hand.

Once you have done the sweeping, break the egg into a crystal glass or clear glass of water.

If the egg shows something that looks like straight pins in the water, that indicates that someone cursed him with something dreadful. If the egg looks all scrambled, it means that he is scared, or something has scared him in the past or that he has been traumatized.

If the egg is clear, that is really clean it means that he does not have any negative supernatural influences at this moment. If it has an appearance of an eye in the yolk, it means he has the evil eye or *mal ojo*.

Regardless of whatever appears in the egg, continue the same ritual for a total of nine consecutive days. After studying the egg, you can dispose of it by flushing it down the toilet. But let me know on a daily basis what you see in the egg.

Let me know immediately if he hears voices, or if he is attacked by a spirit, or has visions or if he has any bad reaction of any kind.

I also recommend that you bathe him in Holy Water from a Catholic Church for the same nine days that you cleanse him with the egg. Let me know if other family members in the same household begin to notice strange or unexplainable things.

Nothing can be more frightening than encountering serious evidence of witchcraft in the form of a doll with needles, *alfileres*, or to "recognize" straight pins within the yolk of an egg that has been used in a cure, or *limpia*.

While actual straight pins have been known to appear in egg yolks, apparently the questioner is talking about parts of the egg that look like pins.

Sympathetic magic is based upon making an association of two unrelated items and the belief that one causes the other.

Witchcraft objects should never be touched with a bare hand and always removed with gloves on. You should always consult a reputable *Curandera* for expert advice.

Making a small fire away from the house and burning the witchcraft dolls is a common remedy, but you must be very careful because the hex will try to "jump," or *brincar*, from the burning doll to a nearby human or animal; thus, transferring and continuing the witchcraft. The gloves which are worn during this process must be burned as well.

CURSED CHILDREN
LOQUITOS

Grandmother, my boyfriend and I have a three-year-old boy who is late in his development. He has had difficulty walking and talking and sometimes he is very quiet for hours. When this occurs, it is like he is locked inside his head.

At other times, he is very hyper and uncontrollable. My boyfriend and I think he will be okay and will develop at his own speed. I know we overprotect him from his cousins.

Now that he is getting to the age where he could go to school, we are thinking of having him evaluated. When we mentioned this to my family, they just laughed and said that he is crazy and will never amount to anything.

We got really mad and off ended about this, and our boy was watching and understands everything, began to yell and cry on the floor. He has feelings, you know?

Then it got worse and they said he might be possessed by an evil spirit. We don't want our child growing up around people who are going to say these bad things about him.

There are many reasons why your child might act the way he does. These behaviors do not mean that there is anything wrong with him, but it is always good to check everything out.

For example, *susto*, or fright sickness, evil eye, or *mal de ojo*, and unclean spirit possession are all conditions that can afflict a child, but they do not mean that he is "crazy."

You should always check with a medical doctor as well. Many children are being diagnosed with attention deficit hyperactivity disorder (ADHD), autism or any other childhood problem, but only a doctor can be sure of what he has if anything at all.

Often, a child who is unable to hear and unable to speak, or who seems to be developing slowly is suffering from some kind of trauma that caused fright, soul loss *susto,* or evil eye, *mal de ojo.*

Think back in his life to when these behaviors began, was there anything that happened to him that you can remember? All these things can be corrected. At the other extreme, there is a possibility that someone is envious of you or your child.

It could even be a family member who has cast a witchcraft spell on him. And yes, it could also be spirit possession, but, once again, all these things can be reversed.

It is a good idea to do two things. Have him cleansed by a reputable *Curandera* and evaluated by a child diagnostician.

Whenever there are signs that something seems wrong with a child, the child should be immediately taken to a medical health care professional for examination, diagnosis, and evaluation. This will help the child and, at the same time, place you at ease.

Also have him spiritually cleansed, but most importantly, never allow your child to be in an environment where people, and especially strangers, are critical of him. If you allow this to continue, then as he grows, what they say about him will form his life's behavioral patterns, whether the comments are true or not. If everyone tells him he is crazy, then he will be crazy. Don't let this happen to your child.

Witchcraft is a major and active force every day in the Hispanic world. Belief in and the practice of witchcraft in the major *Hispanic* communities of the United States is prevalent.

The major migrations of people and news from Latin America available on television and other media, the practice of witchcraft has dramatically escalated in the last few years.

It is important to assist young couples with children to break away from these beliefs so that the new generation of *Hispanics* is not influenced adversely. If the environment is nurturing and not rife with negative news or name calling, bliss allows a child to develop normally and experience a pleasant upbringing.

PROTECT US FROM EVIL
PROTEGIENDO LO NUESTRO

At both our home and at our business we are constantly finding the evidence of witchcraft, and *brujería* objects. Because we are successful, I don't think it will ever end, but is there something we can do to protect our home, our business, and our persons?

As a *Curandera*, I like to practice what I preach. Some of the more popular items that are used for protection for the home, yard, property and business are the *sávila* plant, or aloe vera, which is placed at the entrance of the house or business. It is used to capture negative energies such as envies, jealousies and ill will from enemies as they pass by or enter the home or yard.

As the virtuous plants protect, they absorb negative and evil energies, which usually kills them. So, if your protective plant dies, you know that something evil attempted to get into your home or yard.

A woven strand of garlic heads three to four feet in length is usually placed over the door or near the entrance to the business as well. Never reuse that garlic in cooking; throw it away at the end of every year and get a new one.

Traditionally, and quite popular for the protection of the home, is the use of the *San Ignacio de Loyola* picture, or *estampa*, and the cross made from *palma bendita*, the blessed palm from Palm Sunday which is saved in the home, business and car throughout the year.

Horseshoes, glass containers with water and *tomate marino*, seeds found in the *hierbería*, are also commonly used protective amulets. The Jericho flower with sea shells and red flowers placed in the container will protect the business from bad luck.

For the home, a mixture of white rice, wheat germ and black mustard seed placed in Holy Water and sprinkled outside the home and in the yard will cleanse and protect the property.

Always be certain to sprinkle it over the roof as well. This also "opens the door," *abre camino o puerta*, for the successful sale of the property if that is your wish. Make a written petition and say the appropriate prayers and it will come true.

Florid water, *agua florida*, mixed with ammonia and a little bleach in Holy Water can be used as a floor wash or *despojo* in the home and sprinkled outside the entrance to the home or business for protection.

One of the most common requests people make of a *Curandera*, or a *hierbera* is for protective objects. There are literally thousands of objects and rituals used for this purpose, and each situation is different. Each solution has to consider the unique characteristics of the case.

FOLK PSYCHIATRIST
EL CURA MENTES

Grandmother, I want to thank you for all you have done for me. You have been counseling me for two years now and with your help I have been able to lead a mostly normal life. I was diagnosed with paranoid schizophrenia when I was a teenager and for years, I was not able to attend school or function normally, to hold a job or to have a lasting relationship.

My mother turned to spirituality in order to help me and eventually we were referred to you for help. Even though I take my prescription medications and see a therapist regularly, it was not until I began coming to you for counseling that I was able to keep my mental illness in check. My illness will never leave me but I know that you are protecting me from the evil spirits which surround me.

Even though this torment will be with me for the rest of my life, through your support and prayers I am able to live a normal life. I thank you so much for always being there for me and for protecting me.

Your stability has been remarkable and it should continue as long as you take your medication, see your therapist and place your faith in God. Together we have built a wall of spiritual protection which surrounds you, and your guardian angels will watch over you and keep you from evil. Continue your prayers and always have a candle burning on your home altar. This way you will maintain an impenetrable circle of protection around you.

It is very clear that the *Curandera* provides an important safety net to those who require an ongoing, and sometimes lifelong, cultural component in their treatment. Ari Kiev's book *Curanderismo: Folk Psychiatry* was one of the first studies to deal with *Curanderismo* in a systematic and scientific manner using experiences from a clinical setting. As a psychiatrist who worked in the San Antonio, Texas, area for many years, Kiev theorized that a large percentage of cases presented to *curanderos/as* were directly tied to emotional, psychological and psychiatric issues.

Today *Curanderismo* remains an intriguing mixture of the spiritual, physical and emotional issues and remedies that all people face in the human condition. It is fair to say that *Curanderismo* fills a void in the *Hispanic* culture where psychological and psychiatric counseling are not available in the same way we associate a society of insurance-covered, mental health care access.

There is an ancient history in the Catholic Church, both in Europe and in colonial Mexico, concerning the origins and treatment of mental illness. It was commonly believed that a person's illness was caused by a misdeed or an act against God or a saint.

There are several Catholic saints who are patrons of the behaviorally and mentally ill. Saint Anthony is regarded as the patron of nervous disorders while Saint Cyriacus is the patron of mental disease. Saint Dymphna, is celebrated on May 15th and is generally considered the patron for the insane.

DANCING WITH THE DEVIL
BAILANDO CON EL DIABLO

Finally, we end these fascinating stories with the story of a young girl who danced with the devil. Grandmother the story of the girl dancing with the devil just happened in my town.

There was this girl who was very disobedient and her punishment was to dance with the devil. When my mother told me this story, I was too young to realize that she was training me to be obedient. Since I also love to dance every chance I get, the story fascinated me when I first heard it when I was six.

The story goes something like this: The young girl was very pretty and loved to dance, but she was also very spoiled, *chiflada,* and did not obey her parents. She never obeyed her curfew and worried her parents to death. One time she went to a dance on a Friday night and did not return home until Saturday, and that was the last straw.

She danced all night long until the early morning hours. Since she was very pretty and popular with the boys, her parents worried a lot. She was always able to attract the most handsome boys to her side. This final time, she ignored her parents' warning and they were sick with worry, but once again she ignored their pleas.

Having reached the breaking point, the following weekend her parents did not allow her to go to the Friday night dance. This was to be a very special dance, honoring an engaged couple in the town, *los novios*, but since she was such a disobedient child her parents absolutely would not allow her to attend.

Once again, this wayward girl disobeyed her mother and snuck out of her bedroom window and was off to the dance. When her mother realized that her daughter was gone, she had an uneasy and ominous feeling because she knew that girls like her were punished by a dance with the devil, and not all survive.

The mother wrung her hands and prayed that nothing would happen to her daughter that evening. She could only think of her daughter laughing in her face and saying, "I love to dance!"

The disobedient daughter danced the night away with the local boys. But just before midnight, a handsome stranger entered the dance hall. He was the best-looking young man the girl had ever seen. He was tall with beautiful dark eyes. As he walked towards her, no words were needed; she was lost in his deep eyes as he placed one hand on her waist, and with the other, gently enveloped her hand in his. This was the young man she had been waiting for all her life.

They danced one polka after another, forgetting the witching hour and that she had missed curfew once again. She was enraptured in his spell. The world had disappeared around her. Only the two of them existed.

She didn't want to let go of him, ever. "Will you be here next week, she asked?" He stared deeply into her eyes and then began to laugh. His laugh reverberated from deep within his chest, a dark, unnatural laugh. She tried to step back, but he wouldn't let her go. Instead, his hands became like steel, locking her in place, despite her struggles.

As she chanced to look down, his feet had changed and instead of the shoes that were there before, one foot was shaped like a rooster claw and the other a goat hoof. They were large and red. How had she not noticed them before?

Terrorized, she realized that her dancing partner was the handsome devil, *el diablo guapo*; her mother had warned her about. She screamed loudly not certain of the fate about to befall her.

Some say that she never disobeyed her parents again, others say that she went mad, or *trastornada*. Still, others say that she died engulfed in flames or that she simply disappeared having been taken to hell by the devil. Maybe it was just a dream.

The townsfolk still talk about her to this day, and mothers still tell their daughters to obey and to never dance with handsome devils, pick ordinary boys like their fathers.

It's a fascinating story. This story is almost everywhere there are Mexican Americans or *Hispanics*. This story urges us to obey and that is always a good thing.

My wife also knew a disobedient girl in her town that danced with the devil. In her case, she was consumed by fire and died with the sin of disobeying her parents on her soul. Who knows how she was judged by God.